Counselling Dru
About HIV and

Counselling Drug Users About HIV and AIDS

Geraldine Mulleady
BSc MSc ClinPsychol

OXFORD
BLACKWELL SCIENTIFIC PUBLICATIONS
LONDON EDINBURGH BOSTON
MELBOURNE PARIS BERLIN VIENNA

Blackwell Scientific Publications
Editorial offices:
Osney Mead, Oxford OX2 0EL
25 John Street, London WC1N 2BL
23 Ainslie Place, Edinburgh EH3 6AJ
3 Cambridge Center, Cambridge,
Massachusetts 02142, USA
54 University Street, Carlton,
Victoria 3053, Australia

Other Editorial Offices:
Librairie Arnette SA
2, rue Casimir-Delavigne
75006 Paris
France

Blackwell Wissenschafts-Verlag
Neinekestrasse 4
D-1000 Berlin 15
Germany

Blackwell MZV
Feldgasse 13
A-1238 Wien
Austria

First published 1992

Set by Best-set Typesetter Ltd., Hong Kong
Printed and bound in Great Britain by
Hartnolls Ltd., Bodmin, Cornwall

DISTRIBUTORS

Marston Book Services Ltd
PO Box 87
Oxford OX2 0DT
(*Orders*: Tel: 0865 791155
Fax: 0865 791927
Telex: 837515)

USA
Blackwell Scientific Publications, Inc.
3 Cambridge Center
Cambridge, MA 02142
(*Orders*: Tel: 800 759-6102
617 225-0401)

Canada
Times Mirror Professional Publishing, Ltd
5240 Finch Avenue East
Scarborough, Ontario M1S 5A2
(*Orders*: Tel: 800 268-4178
416 298-1588)

Australia
Blackwell Scientific Publications
(Australia) Pty Ltd
54 University Street,
Carlton, Victoria 3053
(*Orders*: Tel: 03 347-0300)

British Library
Cataloguing in Publication Data

A Catalogue record for this book is available from the British Library

ISBN 0-632-02939-0

Contents

Introduction

The incidence of HIV infection and AIDS is increasing worldwide and is likely to do so for some time, even if a vaccine is developed. It is approximately 40 years since effective drugs against gonorrhoea and syphilis have been available – but these diseases are still prevalent. Although preventative initiatives against HIV infection have been developed in the UK, progress seems painfully slow. I fear that in the area of drug work we manifest the great British characteristic of coping with the problem only after it has become so established that it can no longer be effectively prevented.

According to Jonathan Mann, who was director of the World Health Organization's global programme on AIDS, the pattern of spread which is emerging is one where the heterosexual and maternal routes of transmission predominate. Heterosexual transmission of HIV constitutes the most common route in the world. Among intravenous drug users (IDUs), the sexual route of transmission was often assumed to have less significance than the injecting route. Evidence which questions this assumption is presented here.

Drug users are individuals. Generalisations about what 'they' as a group do can be damaging if this leads to stereotyped assumptions about behaviour. 'They' are us, our partners, parents and children. The use of mood-altering substances or dependency on routines and habits are as much a part of our culture as the air we breathe. How deviant in nature we perceive drug use to be largely depends on our particular culture and our particular society's response to that drug. In the UK, alcohol is seen currently as a socially acceptable drug; heroin is not. A couple of decades ago, cigarette smoking was held to be the sophisticated person's fashion accessory; nowadays, the antisocial aspect of this behaviour has gained prominence.

Initially attention was focused on particular groups – homosexuals, for example – without looking at the possible risk factors themselves within these groups. It is now time to stop talking about 'bridging groups', to stop pointing the finger at people, and to focus on the activities that are known to be associated with HIV transmission. For example, the Federal Drug Administration in the United States has the following recommendations for the exclusion of donors to blood banks: Haitians, immigrants from sub-Saharan Africa, men who have or have had sex with men, prostitutes and their clients, and injecting drug users. Given these preclusions it is reassuring to know that significant advances have been made in the development of a viable substitute for human blood!

The information that we have so far gathered about HIV is neverthless subject to change as time goes on. Research evidence itself is also subject to differing interpretations. The worker has to try to make sense of the facts in order to present them clearly for their clients – here, drug users. This may be difficult both in terms of your time and your training which may not enable you to understand scientific terminology (and jargon) very readily. This does not mean that you need a science degree in order to understand information about the virus, but it does mean that you have to have a commitment to keep your knowledge as accurate and up-to-date as possible. Since there is often an all-too-human tendency to avoid factual information, and as much training in the counselling professions does not familiarise us with scientific terminology, we may feel uncomfortable about discussing these subjects with our clients. This lack can be helped enormously – with a little perseverance and a lot of asking for explanations from people who do understand the 'technical stuff'. The resource list at the end of this book provides a starting point for obtaining more detailed information. Numerous training courses are available, and some good summary journals give a general overview of developments: an example being 'The AIDS Newsletter', published by the London School of Hygiene and Tropical Medicine. They may not provide great detail, but detail may not be required.

The availability of factual information is not the only requirement of the counsellor: Henry *et al.*[1] found that among health care workers the level of formal education was highly correlated with the extent of knowledge about AIDS; it was not, however, correlated with desirable attitudes and behaviours. Therefore, having the necessary information is no guarantee in itself that a person will have an appropriately caring attitude towards people with AIDS and HIV.

A number of factors have been identified as important in terms of what the client perceives as helpful to their situation. These factors have been identified as: advice or specialist knowledge; the understanding given by the counsellor; and the availability of time to talk about self and problems.[2,3] It is probably more productive to see 'counselling' in these terms rather than to attempt a more rigid definition, although some have attempted this, often with little real agreement or consensus.

Those who work with drug users and injecting drug users, collectively referred to as IDUs, do this in a wide range of settings and from a wide variety of backgrounds. Each person working with those affected by HIV will have their own approach and preferred methods of work. A proper understanding of our own beliefs and values is important, as our attitudes influence the counselling work we do. Counselling is not about telling people what to do, it is about enabling clients to make informed decisions about what they want for themselves. There will be cultural and/or religiously determined patterns of behaviour which will lead people to develop attitudes which we may not understand and which may not be conducive to the open discussion of sexual behaviour or to the consideration of such issues as the use of contraceptives to prevent conception in the first place. Thus, we need to be sensitive to a client's background and attitudes before we launch into our own objectives.

Until recently the concept of attracting clients to drug services was a fairly alien one, especially for statutory services. Although one of the indirect effects of HIV has been to highlight this need, not enough is being done to provide services for ethnic minorities and different cultural groups. These groups are frequently under-represented, both in the client group and in the workforce. Practical problems can also emerge if the client's first language is not English and none of the workers in the agency have a relevant second language. More than lip service needs to be paid to equal opportunities within the NHS if these needs are to be addressed.

The main purpose of this book is to provide a broad overview of how the human immune deficiency virus (HIV) can affect the life of the drug user. It sets out to provide some basic information both about the virus and the issues the worker needs to be aware of when counselling drug users. It is suitable either for people who work full-time in the drugs field or those who encounter drug users in non-specialist settings. It is my intention that the book be used as a practical tool for workers who already have an awareness or experience of basic counselling skills. Hopefully, it will serve as an adjunct to these skills. It is not intended as a 'how to' guide to counselling since each worker will have their own style and approach to counselling work. The book itself is based on my own practical experience of counselling in the field of drugs use and HIV at St Mary's Hospital Paddington.

Geraldine Mulleady
January 1992

References

1. Henry, K., Campbell, S. & Willenbring, K. (1990) A cross sectional analysis of variables impacting on AIDS related knowledge, attitudes and behaviours among employees of a Minnesota teaching hospital. *AIDS Education and Prevention*, **2**, (1), 36–47.
2. Murphy, P.M., Cramer, D. & Lillie, F.J. (1984) The relationship between curative factors perceived by patients in their psychotherapy and treatment outcome: an exploratory study. *British Journal of Medical Psychology*, **57**, 187–92.
3. Whale, G. (1987) Distinctive contributions from clinical psychologists? *Clinical Psychology Forum* **8**, 11–14.

Acknowledgements

I would like to thank Jan Souridis for her tireless preparation of this manuscript. Steven Cranfield and John Dunworth for their advice, editorial comments and encouragement, and Nigel Moxham for his enduring patience, support and love.

Chapter 1

The Human Immune Deficiency Virus (HIV) and AIDS-related Illness

Introduction

Acquired immune deficiency syndrome (AIDS) is a disease state arising as a result of infection with the human immunodeficiency virus (HIV). The syndrome is mainly characterised by a reduction of cells in the immune system, the T4 lymphocytes. Damage to the immune system provides the opportunity for various opportunistic infections and tumours to invade the individual. The disease spectrum ranges from asymptomatic individuals with no apparent symptoms to those with disease progression and eventual death either from infection(s) or malignancy.

The immune system

HIV is attracted to particular cells (host cells) in the body. Once inside these cells it can reproduce; in the process it stops the host cell from carrying out its normal function and eventually destroys it. HIV's main target cells are a type of lymphocyte (white blood cell) called the T4 or T-helper cell (or T-helper lymphocyte). The T-helper cells play a crucial role in mobilising our immune system, that is, our body's defence mechanism against disease and illness.

T-cells have been referred to as the leader of the orchestra in our immune system because of their central role in the immune response. There are a range of other types of cells involved in this response, all with specialised functions. The T-helper cell is stimulated to work upon contact with a foreign particle (the antigen), in this case HIV. An antigen is any substance (usually a protein) that, upon contact, can cause an antibody response. On contact with the antigen the T-helper cell goes on to activate other cells in the immune system which eventually destroy the invading particle. The T-suppressor cell is involved in switching the immune reaction off once the job is complete. If the T-helper cell is destroyed as a result of infection with HIV then the whole immune system is affected: an essential link in the chain is missing, with a resultant imbalance in other immune cells involved in the immune response.

It is now recognised that HIV is attracted to a particular protein on the surface of the T-helper cell, the so-called CD4 antigen. This molecule is also found in other cells in the body. As a result some of these cells (listed as follows) are directly affected by HIV:

Macrophages. Part of the immune system which ingests and destroys foreign particles or antigens.
B-cells. Cells which produce essential chemicals in the immune system.
Brain cells. Glial cells in the brain tissue.

The building blocks of life on this planet consist of two main proteins: deoxyribonucleic acid (DNA) and ribonucleic acid (RNA). Normally, the flow of information is from less complex to more complex: less complex organisms like plants tend to be made of RNA; DNA is more complex and makes animal proteins.

A virus is basically a piece of genetic information that requires a living (host) cell in order to reproduce itself. The human immune deficiency virus belongs to a unique family of viruses – retroviruses – which occur in both man and animal.

The retrovirus family reverses this process of replication (hence the term *retro*, meaning backward). They do this by using an enzyme that is unique to their family, reverse transcriptase. (An enzyme is a substance which helps to catalyse chemical reactions in the body.) This enzyme enables viral RNA to make copies of itself out of the host cell's DNA; these RNA copies then leave their host cell and can go on to infect other host cells.

HIV (Fig. 1.1) consists of a protective outer coating, sometimes referred to as the 'envelope'. This is made up of fat and protein (glycoprotein), and the genetic information is contained inside this envelope. One of the reasons why it has proved so difficult to produce an effective vaccine against HIV is that the glycoprotein molecules in the envelope are subject to considerable variation in their format (polymorphism). A vaccine whose mode of action is to recognise and attach itself to the HIV envelope is therefore less likely to be effective.

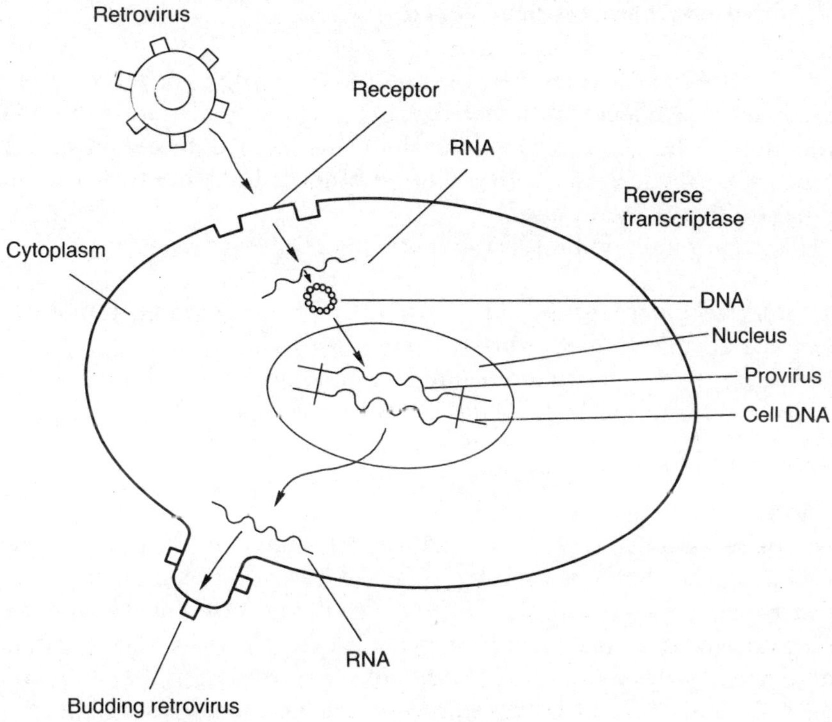

Fig. 1.1 The retrovirus replication cycle.[1]

A second problem with producing an effective vaccine is that HIV lives within the cell itself. Any vaccine, therefore, needs to be able to stop HIV from working without at the same time destroying the human cells in which it lives.

Many if not all the symptoms of HIV infection are caused by the profound damage which it can cause to the immune system; thus the infected person cannot fight off certain infections. A total breakdown of the immune system does not necessarily occur, but the individual becomes vulnerable to infections which can occur as a result of immune suppression as well as to more severe forms of illness which can affect people whose immune system is intact. These infections are described as 'opportunistic' because they take advantage of the person's damaged immunity. Many of the infections are due to re-activation of organisms already present in the individual in a dormant state, or to organisms that commonly occur in the environment and to which we are continuously exposed.

Viral transmission and mutation

In an infected individual, HIV can be found in high concentrations in blood and (in males) in semen since T4-lymphocytes are present in both these body fluids. The virus has also been detected in cervical secretions, saliva, urine, tears, cell-free plasma, bone marrow, cerebrospinal fluid and breast milk.

HIV can be transmitted in the following manner:

- if infected blood gets into the body of another person via transfusion or shared injecting equipment;
- by unprotected sex where semen, vaginal and cervical secretions or blood get into the body of another person;
- from infected mother to baby.

As has been said, HIV antibodies have also been found in saliva in low concentrations as well as in cell-free plasma, urine and tears. There is no evidence that these body fluids act as vectors for transmission.

In explaining transmission factors to clients, reference to the concepts of *quantity*, *quality* and *opportunity* are all useful ones. Firstly, there needs to be a sufficient *quantity* of virus present in the body fluid; secondly, this has to be of sufficient quality, i.e. in a viable form. Thirdly, *opportunity* is required for transmission to occur, i.e. entry into another person via contact with non-skin surfaces like the rectal lining or through the skin via a shared needled syringe.

Whether or not transmission takes place also seems to depend on additional factors such as the following:

- level of trauma or injury;
- re-exposure to the virus;
- the efficiency or integrity of the skin barrier;
- the presence of cells to which HIV is attracted;
- the type of exposure;
- possible genetic factors;
- the phase of infection.

Infectiousness seems to vary over the course of the illness, being high at an early phase following initial infection (the process known as seroconversion), and increasing at the onset of AIDS; it may, however, remain low at other times.

HIV-2

In the mid 1980s a second form of the HIV virus was discovered and found to be highly prevalent in West Africa. There are so far two identified strains of HIV. HIV-2, a second form of the virus, appears to be similar in action and effect to HIV-1. It is also sufficiently different from HIV-1 to mean that most serological tests fail to detect it. HIV-2 has been discovered outside West Africa and this has led many European countries to introduce tests which can detect antibody to HIV-2 reliably. Most laboratories in this country will test simultaneously for both HIV-1 and -2. Thus far, what applies to HIV-1 in terms of the spectrum of AIDS-related illness, seems to apply equally to HIV-2.

Epidemiology

As a counsellor you may be asked by seropositive clients, 'Will I get AIDS?' Reliance on statistics alone to answer this question is unwise, since statistics, are frequently misleading, based as they are on groups of people and not individuals. Furthermore, these groups do not necessarily represent the lifestyle or experience of the client who happens to be in front of you. Another problem is that a client who is given a prediction about their life expectancy may use this as a self-fulfilling prophesy, give up, and thus diminish both the length and quality of their life. This does not mean that the client should be denied access to statistics if they so wish, especially if they are developing illnesses and wish to make plans for their future, but it can be a difficult balance to achieve. So far the average period between exposure to the virus and the development of symptomatic infection is about eight years, but as more data become available and with the development of improved diagnostic and treatment methods, this time period is likely to be extended.

The most recent epidemiological evidence comes from a study of gay men in San Francisco. This is the longest running follow-up study of people with HIV and is an attempt to determine the natural history of the illness in this group. Of the men estimated to have seroconverted to HIV from 1977 to 1980, by 1990 it was reported that 81% had either died of AIDS or developed signs of symptoms; 19% had not yet developed clinical symptoms or signs of HIV-related conditions. Rutherford *et al.* suggest that within 10 years following HIV infection, up to one half of the people infected will develop AIDS and a further quarter to one-third will have some HIV-related illness.[2]

HIV is a slow acting virus; this fact accounts for the time it has taken to learn about the full spectrum of HIV-related disease and why the system for classifying HIV disease and AIDS has been up dated subject to more information becoming available about how the syndrome manifests.

One of the problems with any classification system is that it can be difficult for both clients and non-medical staff to understand. As a result of this many people still use the terminology of the previous classification system, such terms as AIDS-related complex or ARC, for example. The terms 'HIV-related illness', 'HIV disease' or 'AIDS indicator' disease, used in the new classification system, can also be confusing. However, clear understanding of what a client's particular diagnosis means is important as it may have implications for eligibility for medical treatments, state benefits, housing priority and grants from charitable organisations.

The disease spectrum

A number of categories of infection or tumours have been drawn up. The best indicator of immune system damage appears to be the type and severity of infection or tumour that the person develops. A diagnosis will be made on the basis of physical examination and laboratory tests. Not all people infected react to HIV in the same way so they will not necessarily fit neatly into these categories. It should also be borne in mind that this system may be added to or altered as time goes on. Some examples of infections are included in each category, but the list is not exhaustive. In some cases, for example, with thrush or herpes, the severity or site of the infection will determine which classification group is appropriate.

The following classification system for HIV infection is currently used.

Group I – acute HIV infection

Acute seroconversion illness, sometimes a glandular fever or flu-like illness. It does not necessarily occur in all cases. About 10 to 15% of people suffer from this within a few weeks of becoming infected. The symptoms may include fever, malaise, enlarged lymph nodes, headaches and rash. In most cases this resolves spontaneously after several weeks. An HIV-antibody test is negative or equivocal at onset but becomes positive during its course. Otherwise the person feels well and has no other symptoms or signs.

Group II – asymptomatic seropositive

Whether or not they have seroconversion illness, all people pass through a phase that can last months or years when they have no signs or symptoms. It has been broadly estimated that it may take 8 to 12 years after infection for HIV symptoms to occur.

Group III – persistent generalised lymphadenopathy (PGL)

Swollen glands (lymph nodes) in the neck, armpits or groin for more than three months and with no explanation other than the presence of HIV.

A quarter to a third of people who are otherwise without symptoms have enlarged lymph nodes. In the absence of other symptoms, PGL seems relatively benign; the rate of progression to AIDS is not greater than for those at stage II, but it is a very obvious reminder of HIV infection to the individual.

Group IV – HIV with disease

This group is further subdivided and categorised by the Center for Disease Control (CDC) as follows.

a: Constritutional disease

Chronic active viral infection with constitutional symptoms, for example, involuntary weight loss of more than 10%, diarrhoea for at least one month in the absence of other illnesses at the same time. This can be caused directly by HIV or as a result of other gut infections. It can be a very distressing symptom since it becomes so evident to other people that the person is unwell. It should be remembered that the IDUs nutritional neglect is frequently a cause of non-HIV-related weight loss in itself.

b: Neurological disease

This is due to the direct effects of HIV on the brain and nervous system, e.g. dementia. HIV in itself can cause neurological problems. This causes major difficulties because many of the medications currently in use do not cross the blood brain barrier (with the exception of AZT). The direct effect of HIV on the brain is to cause atrophy or loss of brain tissue. This produces a dementia-like syndrome (common in people in their 60s and 70s). The symptoms of this are initially loss of short-term memory and poor concentration, leading to a gradual loss of sensation, incontinence, and problems controlling body movement. It can eventually lead to coma. It is reported to occur in about 25% of people with AIDS. The spinal or facial nerves can be involved and cause peripheral nerve damage – tingling or loss of sensation and movement.

The effects of many drugs may result in poor concentration, transient memory loss and problems with controlling body movement. Drug withdrawal (e.g. from tranquillisers) may also mimic some of these effects. Unless the client is forthcoming about the drugs they are using, this can make an accurate diagnosis much more complicated.

c1: Infections recognised as AIDS (AIDS- defining conditions)

Pneumocystis carinii pneumonia (PCP). This is a bacterial infection to which most of us have been exposed in childhood. By the age of four, 70% of children have developed antibodies to it. If our immune system is intact it causes no problems. This is the commonest type of respiratory infection in AIDS, characterised by a dry cough (non-productive of phlegm), high temperature, tightness of the chest and breathlessness on exertion. It has an acute mortality rate of 35%. It carries a worse prognosis than Kaposi's Sarcoma (see below). It is currently the most common cause of death in IDUs with HIV.

Gut problems. There are many causes of gut problems in HIV infection. One of the most unpleasant is a protozoal infection, cryptosporidiosis. This causes severe watery diarrhoea, colicky pain and malabsorption with marked weight loss. There is no definitive treatment and this means that it is not possible to get rid of the organism that causes it although it is possible to control the symptoms. There can also be direct effects of HIV on the gut. The symptoms of gut involvement in HIV disease are characterised by diarrhoea, abdominal pain and distention with weight loss and fever. Salmonella in people with AIDS can cause blood poisoning, inflammation of the gut, and high fever. It usually results from eating contaminated food, especially undercooked chicken or shellfish.

c2: Symptomatic or invasive disease

Candidiasis (thrush). This is a yeast infection, a common cause of vaginitis in women, especially after antibiotic treatment. When it occurs in the mouth, it is indicative of an underlying defect in the immune system, but it does not by itself constitute a diagnosis of AIDS. However, thrush occurring in the gullet or throughout the body is indicative of a more serious immune dysfunction (i.e. category C1). Thrush can cause discomfort and pain on swallowing and interfere with absorption of food. Oral thrush is considered as an early marker of immune dysfunction and is very common, although other possible causes of thrush must be excluded.

Due to poor dental hygiene many drug users have gum problems such as caries and gingivitis, which also occur in people with immune dysfunction.

Toxoplasmosis. This is caused by a protozoal organism (a single-celled animal). This infection is a common problem in people with AIDS and can cause abscesses on the brain. The individual may have problems controlling body movement or be subject to fits. Symptoms can include fever, headaches, and personality or behavioural changes. The infective agent is commonly found in raw meat and cat feces. It has been shown to have a serious effect on the health of the fetus in pregnant women. People with HIV are advised not to handle cat litter trays without using gloves. Some clinicians estimate that much of the population has already been exposed to toxoplasmosis but it still makes sense, to take precautions. Other brain infections like meningitis and encephalitis may be caused by pathogens such as *cyptococcus*.

Herpes. Herpes simplex lesions commonly occur around the mouth, genitals, anus or gullet. They can occur or recur with disease progression. If herpes occurs in the lung or throat for more than one month, it is included under category C1 – AIDS. Shingles is caused by a related virus, *cytomegalovirus* (CMV). CMV can affect various parts of the body, including lungs, brain, gut and eyes. If it occurs on the retina of the eye it can cause blindness. Prompt treatment is necessary to prevent this.

Tuberculosis. This infection tends to occur early in the course of the illness. It is common among drugs users and may be due in part to pre-existing poor levels of health. In HIV disease it tends to be caused by atypical mycobacteria. It can cause fever, drenching night sweats, shortness of breath, bowel disturbance, fatigue, and swollen lymph glands. It may facilitate the development of other infections such as meningitis or pneumonia. Increasing rates of TB have been observed with the advent of HIV, especially among IDUs in Europe and the USA.[3] This is believed to be caused by reactivation of latent TB infection.[4]

Hairy oral leukoplakia. These are sticky whitish lesions that occur on the sides and undersides of the tongue. They do not require treatment, but are a marker for disease progression.

Salmonella. Recurrent episodes of salmonella infection (a common cause of 'food poisoning') are also included in this category.

d: Malignancies recognised as AIDS

Kaposi's sarcoma (KS). This is a form of skin cancer, most commonly seen in gay men with AIDS, and is rare among heterosexual drug users with AIDS. It is possible that the tumour is caused by a virus that is sexually transmitted and therefore may be one adjunctive factor in infection with HIV. The slightly raised brown or purplish lesions that it causes neither hurt nor itch. They can cause physical problems when they occur inside the body in sites such as the lungs, bowel, stomach or lymph nodes. Certain tumours of the lymph nodes (lymphomas) occur more frequently in people with HIV infection and AIDS.

e: Miscellaneous or other infections

These are indicative of a defect in cell-mediated immunity.

Skin conditions. Skin is commonly affected in HIV disease. It frequently becomes dry and scaly. Skin conditions can cause great distress, especially if they occur on the face (the same applies with KS lesions). The two commonest conditions are seborritic dermatitis – scaling of the facial skin – and folliculitis – severe itchy rash on face, neck and limbs.

Thrombocytopenic purpura (Low platelet count). Platelets are specialised blood cells which play an essential part in the process of clotting. Low platelet count can lead to spontaneous bleeding (usually internal). Initially, this is mostly seen as a distinct tendency to bruising. Before the prevalence of HIV this condition was most commonly seen in young children and middle-aged women.

Diagnosing AIDS

The term 'HIV disease' covers the full range of conditions from initial infection onwards. Some people can die of infections without ever developing AIDS, although they will have symptoms and signs which are suggestive of damage to the immune system. Essentially, no simple progression that most people follow can be defined. An AIDS diagnosis will be made if the person has certain specific tumours or opportunistic infections (viral, fungal, protozoal, bacterial) in more severe forms than normally seen: candida in the mouth, for example, will not constitute an AIDS diagnosis; if it occurs in the gut or lungs, however, then it will. Neurological involvement in the absence of a cause other than HIV is also included.

Diagnostic key

AIDS-related illness: Group IV, a, c2, e and mild forms of b.
AIDS: Group IV, b, c1, d, e and severe forms of a.

The principal AIDS-defining conditions, are as follows:

Infections
Protozoa
- Cryptosporidiosis – with diarrhoea for more than a month
- *Pneumoncystis carinii* pneumonia
- Toxoplasmosis – affecting the brain

Fungi
- Candidiasis (thrush) – affecting the respiratory tract or the oesophagus
- *Cryptococcus* – affecting sites other than the lung

Bacteria
- Mycobacteriosis – TB or related infections of sites other than the lung

Viruses
- Herpes simplex – ulcers for over a month or affecting lungs or oesophagus

- Cytomegalovirus disease – other than in the liver, spleen or lymph nodes; retinitis with loss of vision

Malignancies
- Kaposi's sarcoma
- Lymphoma – primarily lymphoma of the brain, or other non-Hodgkin's lymphoma

Non-infectious, non-malignant conditions
- HIV encephalopathy (dementia) – a disabling failure of mobility and/or physical function for which no other cause can be found

References

1. Jeffries, D. (1986) Virology. In: *The Management of AIDS Patients*. (Eds. D. Miller, J. Weber, & J. Green), London: Macmillan.
2. Rutherford, G.W., Lifson A.R., Hessol, N.A. *et al.* (1990) Course of HIV-1 infection in a cohort of homosexual and bisexual men: an 11 year follow up study. *British Medical Journal* 1990, No. 6762, **301**, 1183–118.
3. Selwyn, P.A., Hartel, D., Lewis, V.A. *et al.* (1989) A prospective study of the risk of tuberculosis among intravenous drug users with HIV infection. *New England Journal of Medicine*, **320**, 545–50.
4. Friedman, I.N., Sullivan G.M., Bevilaqua, R.P. & Loscos, R. (1987) Tuberculosis screening in alcoholics and drug addicts. *American Review of Respiratory Diseases*, **136**, 1188–92.

Chapter 2

Working with Drug Users and HIV

Introduction

When HIV is on the clinical agenda, the worker is frequently the last person to be considered – perhaps because the affect of HIV on the client so commands our attention. However, if the worker is to function with consistency and to a high standard, it is essential that we address the basic tenets of our training, practice and support systems. It is something of a cliché that we must care for ourselves before we can care for others but this is especially true in the drug field where too often the worker is thrown in at the deep end and expected to cope. It is for this reason that the chapter that follows considers some of the issues that particularly affect the worker who is involved in HIV and drugs counselling.

Confidentiality

In the UK HIV is treated in relation to the law as a sexually transmitted disease (although it can be transmitted in other ways) and is dealt with under the 1974 Venereal Diseases Act. Regulation 2 provides that:

> 'Every health authority shall take all the necessary steps to secure that any information identifying an individual obtained with respect to persons examined or treated for any sexually transmitted disease shall not be disclosed except for the purpose of communicating the information to a doctor or someone working under his direction in connection with the treatment of persons suffering from the disease or the prevention of its spread'.

This means that information about an individual's HIV antibody status is confidential and should not be disclosed to any other person without the prior consent of the client. The General Medical Council lists the circumstances for doctors where confidentiality can be breached. These include: cases of suspected child abuse; disclosure in the public interest such as investigation of a serious crime by the police; sharing information with other health professionals involved in the care of the patient; and disclosure by order of a court of law. It is assumed that these regulations apply to both AIDS and HIV.

In other countries, medical practitioners may have even greater freedom, as, for example, the decision of the Irish Medical Council that they 'may, in all the circumstances of the case, consider it is a duty to inform the spouse or other partner' that a patient is HIV positive. This kind of decision is likely to deter people from coming for help and may serve to push the problem underground. It is an undeniably awful position to be in where you see a couple and know that one of them is positive and that they have not yet told their partner. I hasten to add that this situation is rare and usually the HIV positive partner does disclose his or her status. However, until this disclosure comes about it can be very difficult for the worker.

Drug services have always been fairly enlightened about client confidentiality but an increased awareness is now necessary. You should be aware of your own unit's policy if it has one; if it does not, then it should be encouraged to develop one. However, the reality of how these policies work is often very different from how they appear on paper and they can run into serious difficulties in practice. A good working policy is one that is clear to staff and clients at the outset. In the process of developing these policies, it is useful to run through a couple of 'difficult' scenarios, incidents that may arise where the staff have to react without advance preparation, in other words to think on their feet.

Confidentiality exists to protect the clients' rights. If they feel that this is the case then they will be more likely to come and use your service. Respecting confidentiality is not the same as keeping secrets with the client. If you work in a team it is impossible to hold secrets on behalf of the client and at the same time be fully supported by your team. If you work with more than one staff team then you and the team need to be clear about the information you are expected to share for the benefit of the client. Clarify the principle of team confidentiality with a client at the outset in order to avoid misunderstandings. If you can be up front about your 'team confidentiality' policy then your position is less likely to be compromised. It is useful to have written consent from the client, as a basic requirement, before communication is entered into with another agency where disclosure of the client's

HIV status is necessary. Clear channels of communication mean that the client often receives a better service.

Professional boundaries

Drug workers, possibly more than any other health-related specialist area, come from a wide variety of backgrounds, professional disciplines and training. The most basic difference between ourselves and our clients is that (usually) we are paid and have chosen to do drug work. We need to be able to set limits or boundaries of acceptable behaviour for ourselves and a client, an awareness that these boundaries will be tested, and sensitivity to the feelings that boundaries can evoke in a client. How do we respond to rules? The IDU's use of testing or challenging behaviour may be to gauge the counsellor's ability not only to cope with problems but also to measure the counsellor's capacity to cope with their feelings of inadequacy and dependency. Too often we see workers who are afraid to set boundaries and limits and who get their fingers burnt and then back off and become cynical and distrustful. We have only ourselves to blame if we allow the opportunity for 'manipulation' to arise. It is those who allow abuse of their 'kindness' who are in part responsible for negative image and stereotyping of IDUs. Stereotyping can just as easily (and unfairly) be applied to the drug worker, as follows:

The street cred. Likes to view themselves as radical; understands their clients better than other agencies; nearly always anti-establishment.

The bigot. Tends to work in more 'establishment' settings; usually operates a rigid appointment system and is frequently heard to voice the opinion that most drug users are psychopaths.

The professional. Well balanced, highly motivated and valued by their employers; makes appropriate use of support and supervision. Usually athletic.

The burnt out. Any of the above after approximately two years!

Boundary setting does not mean that one should be unnecessarily guarded; it should be seen as keeping the client/worker relationship as safe and intact as possible. Limit setting is the foundation of a professional approach to such counselling work.

As part of boundary setting, we should not tell clients our own problems (unless in a co-counselling context), nor moan to them about other workers or units. If we do, we should ask ourselves who, in the long run, benefits from this? Instead, if the worker has a problem, say, with another unit, this should be dealt with in staff supervision and ideally worked through with the agencies in question.

On a very basic level, boundary setting extends to setting time limits. Frequently clients will say something very important at the end of their interview, often in the form of a throw-away statement. You have the practical consideration that you have to finish the session and the dilemma that the client has just said something very significant – probably a comment on how they have been feeling all the time. It is important to acknowledge this; often people drop statements at this stage because they know the session is ending and it is fairly safe to make the statement. It could also be a challenge to the need to end the session. There is a big difference between a 15- to 20-minute over-run on an occasional basis and a one hour session developing into one of two hours. How you view this, of course, will depend on the way you work and on your work setting.

To use a drop-in setting as an illustration of the above, here it is more difficult to use an appointment system and the nature of the work that emerges is unpredictable. In this situation you may have clients who choose to see you when in crisis without any guarantee that they will come back again. A choice has to be made between dealing with the problem there and then or negotiating with the client to look at it another time. You may choose to ask the client the reasons they chose to make the statement at the end of the session, acknowledge its importance and the fact that you would like to talk about that when you have more time in order to make sure that you can give the issue the time it deserves, and admit that there is no time at the present to devote to it because of other work commitments you have.

It is likely that some drug using clients will require a higher level of advocacy than is routinely required. The long-term goal of counselling is to help the client learn to help themselves and put control back in their lives. In the face of the crises that the IDU can present with, there is a risk of losing sight of this. Again, in the long run, who benefits from the dependent relationship that can develop between client and worker? '. . . was it that she wished so instinctively to help, to give, that people might say of her, "O Mrs Ramsey! Dear Mrs Ramsey . . . Mrs Ramsey, of course!" and need her and send for her and admire her? Was it not secretly this that she wanted,'. . . . From *To The Lighthouse* by Virginia Woolf.

The keyworker principle

A drug user who has HIV or AIDS will inevitably come into contact with a number of different agencies and workers – an ideal situation for snarled up communications. In addition, the client may 'shop around' between the different agencies because they may find a service that is better suited to their needs at the time. Their decision at such a time is often related to the service that can offer the most practical help on the least challenging basis.

One of the added implications of multi-agency involvement is that it will be difficult at times to operate a keyworker principle unless you elicit the co-operation of both the client and the other agencies involved. As is frequently the case, these different agencies do not always have regular or clear routes of communication.

A possible reason for this may be the agency's confidentiality policy or the IDU's decision that they do not want other agencies to be involved. A less dignified reason is the sometimes competitive attitude that agencies and workers can manifest in terms of their ability to attract and hold on to clients affected by HIV. We may work in the 'caring' professions, but none of us leave our egos at home. This unhelpful attitude may be exacerbated by a funding situation which is increasingly reliant on recruiting drug users affected by HIV. However, if you are able to initiate and maintain communication with other workers and agencies, provided this is what the client wants, it can be beneficial to the client by co-ordinating appropriate care and cutting down on duplication of effort.

As a drug worker you may have or develop a long-standing relationship with the client and therefore be in a key position to play a co-ordinating role, but you may also find your role marginalised by more 'mainstream' services.

The role of staff with personal experience of drug use

Many drug workers who come from relatively user friendly settings have commented that IDUs frequently assume that the staff are themselves ex-drug users and therefore understand them better and know what they are going through. Although in most work settings staff members are not ex-users, those who are may be in a position to use their previous experience very powerfully. It is up to the individual whether or not they decide to use their own experience of drug taking in their work with clients. If they choose to do so, and are not simply exploited by the other staff, they can act as role models and so have a crucial role to play. A balance needs to be achieved: being an ex-user is not a badge of office, nor should it be used as one. The same can be said for workers who are on long-term maintenance. One problem that should be acknowledged from the start is that drug workers do jobs which are stressful and demanding, often breaking new ground. These challenging positions are often underpinned by unpredictable funding; in addition, they are sometimes experimental in nature, often lack adequate supervision and support, and can thus expose the non-user and ex-user alike to strains that are quite intolerable.

Ex-users may be particularly vulnerable if they have not had the opportunity to gain professional training or if they over-identify with clients. It is crucial that they have access to and receive regular support and supervision and that the opportunity for training and further development exists. If the requirement is that workers be drug free, some ground rules should be agreed beforehand. An example would be minimum periods of abstinence, such as two years drug free, before staff are exposed to outreach work in drug using communities. Consideration may be given to the initial placement of the ex-user in a less stressful position in order that they have the opportunity to become established before they are exposed to working with active drug users.

Although each individual worker from this group will present with a unique history and set of circumstances, the agency needs to give some thought to difficult questions such as the following:

- how to accommodate workers who have AIDS and whose performance may ultimately be adversely affected by illness;
- how to cope with workers whose personal drug use means that they cannot sustain a minimum acceptable level of job performance;
- how to cope with workers who may be compromising the agency by engaging in illegal drug use;
- what position to take on illegal drug use when this is likely to expose our double standards about the consumption of legal drugs – especially alcohol, excessive use of which is just as likely to adversely affect the worker's level of job performance.

Coping with failure

If as drug workers we find that the client does not change or follow our advice, how do we deal with disappointment, frustration and concern?

When the client does not show demonstrable change, this inevitably raises our anxiety, both in terms of the risk of the client acquiring or transmitting infection and also by the fact that we may start to question our own ability as counsellors.

Both the worker and the client can engage in rationalisation in order to cope with the demands that HIV puts upon them. According to Wilson,[1] initially the IDU may show resistance and engage in manoeuvres that create distance in order to protect themselves from involvement and to avoid getting close to and trusting the worker. The educative component of HIV counselling makes the client feel bad because the client may know that they will not act on the advice given. This can lead the client to feel bad about themselves and suffer from enhanced feelings of inadequacy. They may cope with this by the following methods:

Denial. 'The test result was wrong'.
Rationalisation. 'It didn't happen to my friend so it won't happen to me'.
Avoidance. The client does not come to the sessions at all or comes totally stoned.

The counsellor, in turn, can be affected in exactly the same way.

Rationalisation. 'This is an unmotivated client'.
Displacement. 'If only the other workers involved with this client would get their acts together'.
Avoidance. 'This client needs to be referred elsewhere'.

How do we cope with clients who will not change? It is easy to blame the client entirely for lack of change but we should attempt to assess the change that the client is capable of making in the context of their circumstances at the time. Are there practical barriers? relationship barriers? lifestyle barriers (i.e. time spent out scoring/stealing)? religious or cultural barriers? Can we work with these? We need to start by examining the reasons for the resistance that the client may have.

If necessary we should move to parts of the IDU's life where some change is possible and enable them to achieve this by moving the goalposts and shelving the issue for some time in the future when the client may be more receptive. Whatever we do we cannot control people's lives. At best we can increase their options so that they can exercise a wider range of choices for their own lives. Creativity in approach is called for in combination with allowing the client to set the pace. There are also important differences between initial change and being able to sustain change. In a developing relationship, for example, the couple may see less need for safer sex as issues of trust become more important to them.

In drug work it is often difficult to see any positive change in the lives of some of our more chaotic clients. Having a fairly broad definition of what constitutes progress can help to minimise this. Many drug workers would welcome the opportunity to undertake more 'in depth' therapeutic work with their clients. The reality (at least initially) is that the client is more likely to present because he or she needs help with practical problems such as obtaining a prescription, housing, welfare and rehab admission. It is rare to find that the client's therapeutic needs are their first priority.

Coping with stress

Clients frequently present us with challenges to our competence and when HIV is added to this equation it is not difficult to see where stress management becomes important for both worker and client.

One aspect of drug work that can be annoying is the patronising reaction of others to finding out that this is the work you do. The 'I don't know how you can work with these people' comment, for example. The point is simply that we have *chosen* to work with 'these people'. Drug work, though rewarding, is stressful: we perceive it to be so. In a stress assessment of staff at St Mary's syringe exchange and drug dependency unit, most staff answered 'yes' to the question 'Do you think your job is more stressful than those of your friends and acquaintances who have different jobs.'

Staff support is a basic essential. We get to know our clients over a long period of time. It is not easy to cope with sudden deaths from overdoses or to see our clients' physical decline and death as a result of AIDS. We are not always strong or consistent in our responses. In order to use staff support appropriately, we need to admit to our weaknesses. People who work in the caring professions frequently build walls around themselves and deny that they are vulnerable to emotions like hurt, anger, dislike and pain. This is often the reason why staff support groups fail. Fears for our own safety may emerge, particularly early on in our exposure to HIV work. We may find ourselves evaluating or re-evaluating our own risk behaviours. These factors can all increase the pressures we feel at work. Increased resources may be required in order to fund support, but it should be remembered that these support measures come under the heading of basic necessity rather than luxury and should be built into any job. It is necessary to share our feelings with other people. There are different types of support and supervision and you need to be clear that what is provided is appropriate for your needs. The following list outlines some of the benefits:

- to learn from them and for them to learn from us;
- to share difficulties and maintain perspective;
- to generate a range of solutions;
- to enjoy and validate successes;
- to help workers identify symptoms of stress and anxiety.[2]

In addition, there is frequently a distinct difference between support and supervision. Managerial supervision is generally provided by someone to whom the worker is accountable and addresses issues of policy and working practice. Unless you have a very trusting relationship with your manager you are unlikely to want to tell them that you feel inadequate or cannot cope. Some additional built-in support system is necessary. Clinical supervision may be provided 'in house' but outside facilitators may also be used. This will tend to address the style and content of client-based work and how the worker and client are affected by this. Some overlap between support and supervision is likely to occur in this setting. How much will depend on whether it is in a one-to-one or group setting, and whether it is provided in house, by peer supervision, or by an outside facilitator. These factors will influence the extent of any additional support that is required. Team support and supervision will be affected by staff hierarchies and different roles. Some workers will be in individual therapy where work issues will be touched on.

Some agencies use facilitators to explore the dynamics of the workers' interaction and how personalities/events in the workplace affect this dynamic. This can provide support, but can also be threatening for the staff, and while this type of supervision can help to sort out team problems, the facilitator really needs to know how to contain potentially explosive situations and to diffuse them effectively, to enable staff to leave the group without feelings of bitterness or unfinished business. Facilitators do not necessarily need to be 'bought in'; it may be possible for someone in house who has expertise and competence in the subject to do this.

What is sufficient and acceptable support for one worker may not be so for another. The type of support that works for each of us is obviously a very personal thing, but it is not something that should be left to the worker to sort out without agency backing. The range of choices will depend on the organisation of each agency and their financial resources.

Stress management techniques

A certain level of stress or demand is necessary in order for us to function at optimum levels. However, when demands overtake our resources for coping, we begin to suffer from symptoms of stress. It pays to recognise these in yourself, as well as the events that can precipitate them. There are numerous ways of coping and an extensive literature on the subject. Briefly, without going into inappropriate detail here, the following are some of the ways people can learn to cope:

- stress monitoring and diary keeping;
- sharing feelings with others;
- problem solving techniques;
- avoidance;
- seeking social support;
- seeking information;
- use of appropriate social skills;
- reframing negative or irrational thoughts into rational ones;
- tension reduction and relaxations methods;
- structuring the problem;
- assertive responses;
- maintaining good physical health;
- religious beliefs or strong value systems;
- denial that the problem exists;
- taking drugs or alcohol;
- confidence and control;
- good levels of self esteem.

Obviously some of these ways of coping are not particularly helpful or constructive in all situations. The easier you can fit an adaptive stress reducing strategy into your daily routine, the more likely you will be to sustain it. You will find that if you 'practise what your preach' you will get the message across to your clients with considerably more conviction.

According to George[2] where these techniques apply specifically to work settings we should attempt to do the following:

- monitor hours and keep to job description activities;
- see our limitations;
- seek support, advice, experience;
- refuse requests without feeling guilty;
- forgive ourselves for mistakes;
- express our emotions;
- get sufficient sleep and relaxation;
- allow time for play and entertainment;
- pay attention to diet and exercise;
- develop and monitor social networks;
- set aside time for spiritual needs.

Ensure caring for ourselves as we try to care for others. An example of this last item is where bereavement work is concerned: In this situation it is important to recognise that we cannot satisfy everybody's needs, and we cannot remove the pain of loss, both our own and those left behind. We may be going through events in our own lives which render us unable to cope with bereavement work and in that case we should avoid it if possible. We may not want to do bereavement work. We may come to a stage where we have suffered too many losses and cannot cope with any more. We may come to a stage where we say to ourselves we have done well to work in the area for a while and recognise it is time to move on.

References

1. Wilson, J. (1988) Prevention of infection – the role of counselling. Women and AIDS Conference, Post House Hotel, Edinburgh.
2. George, H. (1990) Coping with dying and bereavement. Training course notes, Leicester: The Association for Psychological Therapies.

Chapter 3

Promoting Behaviour Change in Injecting Drug Users

Introduction

There are an estimated 50 000 heroin users in the UK. Unfortunately, we are not even sure of the exact figures. A relatively small proportion of heroin and other drug users are in contact with drug treatment agencies of any kind. Much research energy has been devoted to trying to find out the reasons why people develop drug problems. Almost all of this work challenges the existence of what are ususally termed global personality characteristics.[1] The quality of drugs research might also be improved by establishing closer working links between psychological and anthropological research methods. In the following chapters some of the issues that particularly affect the worker who is involved in HIV and drug counselling are considered.

The aetiology of drug dependence

Early initiation into drug use and higher levels of injecting have been associated with problems in the family environment. These include structural factors (e.g. separation, divorce, single parent households), and functional factors (e.g. poor communication and absence of harmony and warmth in the home).[2,3] Of 150 heroin users attending three London treatment agencies, Sheehan *et al.*[4] found that the IDUs were disadvantaged with respect to education and employment and often had a difficult family background. Social environment seems to play an important part: in many studies the influence of peers, especially older siblings and early sexual partners, were found to be even more powerful than family influences in predicting adolescent drug use, although the effects of each kind of influence in itself was nevertheless significant.[3,5] At St Mary's Hospital, many of the clients attending the drug clinic were introduced to injecting heroin by an older sibling.

The importance of peer influences in HIV transmission and syringe sharing goes without question. There is relatively little research on drug users who do not attend drug agencies, and also scant information on the experimental or recreational users of drugs such as cocaine and amphetamines. Cocaine and crack use have received more detailed research attention in the United States.

Crack use has been associated with sexual disinhibition. Crack use has also been found to be related to increased incidence of syphilis, gonorrhoea and chancroid, associated with the so-called 'sex for drugs' phenomenon. With cocaine's shorter lived high, drug users inject themselves repeatedly until their supply of drug is finished – thus they inject more frequently than if using heroin alone.[6] Pharmacological interventions for the amphetamine and cocaine user have mainly consisted of the use of tricyclic antidepressants for withdrawal symptoms, although drugs such as disipramine chloride and dopaminergic agents are being investigated.[7,8]

Usage patterns

The *experimental* drug user can be defined as someone who may only use on a limited number of occasions with his or her peer; *social* users are those who use drugs only in certain situations in the appropriate company/circumstances; the *recreational* user may not rely as much on the peer approval factor and will use drugs to enhance enjoyment.[9] Obviously, there is considerable overlap between these groups. The adverse effects of the drugs taken will go some way towards determining whether or not the experimental user will go on to become a social or recreational one. Other factors include the type of drugs available, previous drug experience, financial resources, availability of less toxic drugs such as cannabis, and any initial experience of injecting.

The desire to join in when others are in the process of being initiated into drugs can result in sharing of both drugs and injecting equipment. Newcomers are unlikely to have the appropriate injecting equipment or the technique to inject; it is therefore probable that the novice will begin injecting in the presence of others and share equipment with those teaching the 'art' of injecting.

Recreational users continue to use drugs mainly because they enjoy the effects of the drug. Their drug use will also be determined by availability, price and setting as well as their contacts for supplying a particular drug. Little is known about how the recreational user perceives him or herself, what their knowledge levels with regard to HIV are, and what educational messages they perceive to be relevant to them. Dixon[9] advocates the importance of user groups in order to establish links with the 'invisible' or recreational user. Recreational users will need to develop a sense of ownership of the educational materials because there will be a tendency not to identify with messages aimed at regular drug users.

Where *regular* drug users are concerned, it is worth noting from the St Mary's study that the average duration of drug use before contact with a treatment agency was five years. The educational messages about HIV that users receive before this will be likely to come through the contact with general health care providers. This factor makes HIV prevention an issue for a much wider range of people than drug workers. The experimental user's access to information is very haphazard. The first experience of injecting is almost always a social one. The experimenter's knowledge of safer injecting techniques is likely to be scant and to depend on that of the people they are injecting with. These people in turn may not be perceived by the experimenter as being 'risky' to share works with. Apart from the risk via shared injecting equipment, they may also be more likely to engage in unsafe sex and may be more at risk as a result of the effect of the drug on their behaviour and judgment; there is, for instance, a relationship between drugs and alcohol consumption and unsafe sex.[10] Risk taking is often accepted as part of human development during adolescence and, as part of this process, illicit use of drugs is often embarked on during late adolescence. Experimenters are at high risk of HIV exposure in areas where the background level of infection among IDUs is high. Low HIV prevalence locally will be an important factor as it will influence whether or not people see HIV infection as a likely consequence for them.

The term '*problem drug use*' refers to drug use that results in social, psychological, physical or legal problems associated with dependence, intoxication, or regular excessive consumption.[11] The worker may decide that an individual's drug use constitutes problem use. However, the individual's own perception may differ significantly. It is usually the individual's perception that is the pertinent factor with regard to their obtaining and accepting help with their drug use.

Poly drug use, where more that one drug is used, is common among regular users and a wide range of substances may be taken. Research has indicated that users can adjust their consumption in line with such external factors as price and availability,[12,13] which will vary from one location to another. For example, benzodiazepines are very commonly used by IDUs. Temazepam, for example, can alleviate some of the symptoms of withdrawal from opiates. It can be injected and taken in conjunction with heroin; some users report that it contributes to the 'high'. Such a drug can be obtained fairly easily and is not overly expensive on the so-called 'grey' market (illegally distributed prescribed drugs). Apart from its hypnotic effect, it has been observed to have the effect of increasing agitation and irritability among some users. According to Klee,[14] Temazepam use is associated with higher levels of both syringe sharing and casual sexual contacts, although this may not be a causal effect of the drug, but associated instead with the predisposition of the individual user towards risk-taking behaviour.

For the reasons given above, drug workers need to take into account the whole range of drugs the client may use and their combinations from the perspective of their possible impact on risk-taking behaviour. There will be considerable variability in the individual's response to certain drugs and it will also depend on the following: the amount used; tolerance level; reason for using it; and method of administration. Some people, for example, become drowsy and detached on heroin use; some become more active. Thus it is not yet clear if it is the individual's pre-disposition to risk taking, their individual response to the drug, the drug's detrimental effect on judgment, or the situation/contextual variables, that leads to risk taking. For many IDUs, risk taking is accepted as part of their everyday lives, but not all of these risks may be taken willingly.

The effect of drug use on the immune system is not yet clear. One American study found that abstinence and reduced drug use decreased the likelihood of HIV progression. However, several other studies have failed to show a significant effect.[15,16]

Risk reduction and harm minimisation

Abstinence from drugs is not the only goal of drug work. It is equally legitimate to help make a person's continued drug use safer for them or to offer treatment options where stabilisation of drug use is the goal. When someone has had a drug problem for a number of years, it should be taken that progress is obviously going to be slow and erratic in nature.

If goals are set for our clients that are unrealistically high, then it is easy for both client and worker to become discouraged. Realistic harm minimisation with goals set in agreement with the client can serve to reduce this. Harm minimisation is defined as any change which, on an individual and at a social level, minimises the harm associated with drug use. Risk reduction is encompassed by this and is defined as any measure designed to reduce the risk of transmission of HIV through both drug use and sexual behaviour. As a result of successful risk reduction, drug services are then free to develop strategies to enable them to work with drug users at a wider range of stages in the IDU's career. Some risk reduction strategies are listed below:

- abstinence;
- using but not injecting;
- using but injecting with sterile equipment;
- using but not sharing;
- using and still sharing.[17]

Risk assessment

Before offering advice on risk reduction, it is necessary to assess what risk behaviours (if any) the client is currently engaged in. There are two types of assessment that can be carried out with the client. Risk reduction may specifically address the risks associated with HIV transmission. Harm minimisation may examine the client's situation in a wider context and the two are not mutually exclusive. A broader framework for risk assessment will enable both client and worker to pinpoint more clearly areas of need and improvement in their overall situation.

An assessment can vary between a one-off guide to the priority areas which require intervention to a detailed history taking that can take some time to complete. It should not be so detailed a procedure that it increases the IDU's waiting time before any intervention can take place. The particular emphasis of the assessment will depend on the setting in which it is carried out and the services on offer; this may also have an impact on the worker's comfort or otherwise at having to ask particular questions. The issues involved in sexual history taking are covered in the section on sexual risk reduction. It is probably the case that the drug worker has difficulty in asking questions about the client's sexual behaviour. The worker in the STD clinic on the other hand will see sexual history taking as a completely routine procedure, but may have a few problems asking questions about the client's drug use. The areas covered in risk assessment can include: sexual behaviour; drug use and injecting behaviour; and general health. A wider assessment may include information on emotional/psychological health, finance, family/relationships, employment status, housing and legal problems.

A problem-solving framework (Table 3.1) can be useful in order to break down each problem and develop possible solutions that the IDU and worker can action. In this way the worker can check up on any immediate and longer term action they need to take. Some workers use scales which can be re-done at intervals to assess progress and problem areas that are static. Factors such as regular employment, adequate housing and family support can be useful predictors of stability.

Injecting behaviours

A syringe or hypodermic syringe is a device for injecting or withdrawing fluid be means of pressure or suction. The term 'syringe' is therefore a collective one for both barrel, plunger and needle. The user's common collective term for the syringe (barrel and needle) is 'works'. Some syringes have fixed needle and barrel while in others the needle, barrel and plunger are separable. It is necessary to clarify the local terminology as in some instances the syringe may be interpreted to be the barrel and plunger only. There are also anecdotal reports that IDUs may interpret not sharing to mean not sharing needles and avoid doing this while they continue to share the barrel and plunger.

The mechanism whereby the syringe comes into contact with blood may take the following sequence: the drug to be injected will be in solution. In the case of street heroin it will be mixed with water on a metal spoon or metal bottle cap (the cooker); added to this will be a dissolving agent such as citric acid or vitamin C powder, lemon juice or vinegar. Some forms of heroin, such as Pakistani heroin, require heating in order to complete dissolution. Chinese heroin, which is not widely available now, dissolves without heating. Amphetamine users generally dissolve their drugs in cold water if they are going to inject. If needle and syringe are sterilised there is no possibility of contaminating the cooker. However, infected blood can be pushed out of the needle and syringe and into the cooker in the process of drawing up the drug solution. Even if the cooker is heated, the temperature reached may not be high enough to sterilise it and its contents. The cooker will be heated using matches, a cigarette lighter, and sometimes by lighting the alcohol swabs provided for cleaning the skin surface

Table 3.1 Client assessment.

	Risk assessment	Solutions	
	Current situation	Immediate action	Long-term action
Drug use	No script; wants one; re-uses works. Adequate syringe cleaning. No lending or borrowing equipment in the past six months. Buys works from chemist. Good injecting techniques. Good veins.	Introduce to local syringe exchange and services they offer.	Refer for treatment at DDU.
Sexual behaviour	Steady relationship with user (2-years' duration). Partner knows about HIV status; remains untested. Does not have safer sex.	Willing to bring partner to next session. Discuss safer sex.	

Lifestyle assessment

Health care	HIV+; no symptoms. No medical check as yet. No GP.	Appointment at STD clinic.	Find GP.
Finance	Claims social security. Eligible for community care grant? Bills up to date so far.	Appointment with welfare rights worker.	Liaison re funding applications.
Legal	On probation. No outstanding charges. One prison sentence five years ago.		Contact probation re any training or support group initiatives.
Employment	Unemployed. Dealing. Never had a job. Left school 15. No qualifications. Cannot read.		Interested in literacy classes.
Housing	Council accommodation; 2 bedrooms. Satisfied, but has little furniture.	Welfare rights worker; may benefit from supporting letter.	Lives on 9th floor; may not be suitable if mobility problems develop.

prior to injection. The solution is drawn up into the syringe through a filter placed in the cooker. The filter or 'cotton' is usually a small piece of cotton wool or the filter tip of a cigarette. It is used to strain out undissolved impurities and is often saved and later on washed with water to extract any remains of the drug.

The user then has to find a vein, or may inject into skin or muscle. In order to ensure that they have found a working vein, they will have to draw a little blood into the solution in the syringe. If the vein is suitable (i.e. has not collapsed and is big enough to inject into), then the drug is injected. The drug user will usually want to flush out any drug that remains in the needle and neck of the syringe. In order to do this, they will have to draw blood into the syringe and flush it back again. Thus the needle and syringe will contain small quantities of blood.

If another person injects with the same equipment without attempting to remove this blood, then they risk injecting this mixture into their own bloodstream. If this blood contains HIV, then there is a potential route for transmission of the virus. Flushing does not take place with subcutaneous injections, 'skin popping', but similar HIV transmission risks must be assumed to exist here also.

In HIV transmission, the drug which the user chooses to inject is not the crucial factor; it is the method of administration. A whole range of drugs are injected, whether or not they were designed for that specific purpose: Palfium, amphetamines, cocaine, Temazepam and Diconal are all used. Heroin can be mixed with a number of other drugs barbiturates, for example, and cocaine, as well as 'cutting' agents such as glucose. It has been demonstrated that a significant proportion of the drug users investigated so far are able to reduce their HIV risk behaviours in relation to drug use provided they have the means of doing so through supply of clean injecting equipment and relevant information.

Some studies report that, essentially, all IDUs engage in needle sharing during some period of their drug using careers.[18] Sharing may not be attributed either to ignorance about the consequences of that behaviour or about HIV-prevention. Sharing is often directly related to peer group behaviour, attitudes conducive to sharing, economic motivation to share, not owning injecting equipment, and fatalism about developing AIDS. The prevalence of HIV in the local population will also influence the perception of risk of HIV infection. But as Blattner *et al.* discovered, the more often you inject the more likely you are to be seropositive.[19]

Consistently, the main reason given for sharing seems to be lack of availability of works.[20,21] There are still substantial numbers of users who may share if and when the circumstances call for it, despite the known risk of HIV, and this possibility should be discussed with clients.

In the Central London area where I worked previously, shooting galleries (places where people go specifically to inject drugs) appeared to be rare, although there were anecdotal reports of their existence. People were more likely to be in their own homes when they injected and, in these circumstances, sharing occurred if there was insufficient equipment to go round everyone present. Occasionally, IDUs will inject drugs at the dealer's house so that they are not in possession of drugs when they leave. If they have no works then they will use what is available at the dealer's. Dealers can thus be key people in peer-education, risk reduction, and the distribution of clean syringes.

'Frontloading' is one example of syringe use where, technically, sharing does not occur because it is the drug which is being shared between separate syringes. With this procedure the drug solution is drawn up into one syringe. The plunger is taken out of the other and some of the contents of the first is squirted into it. Although syringe sharing does not occur, if either syringe is contaminated with blood, there is still a risk.

Because of the publicity that syringe sharing has received, the client may be reluctant to discuss syringe sharing issues, dismissing it as 'something they don't do'. Firstly, it is necessary to clarify the difference between *lending* works to others and *borrowing* works from others. Lending works to someone else is sometimes not seen as sharing – the IDU no longer shares themselves, but may allow others to use their works after them. If the client is reluctant to discuss the subject as it applies to them, it may help to de-personalise it by asking, 'if someone were injecting, under what circumstances do you think sharing might occur? How would someone cope with that situation in order to reduce the risks?' Sometimes this can lead to a discussion about the client's communication skills, cleaning methods, and so on.

It is necessary to be sensitive to the conditions and practices of drug use which exist in your local community. The drugs used, the route/s of administration, the availability of sterile equipment, the prevalence of HIV, sharing practices and services will vary from place to place.

In order to provide appropriate advice about reducing risk through drug use, it can be useful to obtain further information from the client. How much information you require and in what sequence you gather it will depend on the context in which you work. It may include the following:

- do you inject?
- how frequently?
- what drugs do you usually inject?
- would you be able/willing to consider safer methods of ingestion, e.g. smoking/sniffing?
- what drugs do you inject occasionally, e.g. Diconal, Temazepam?
- what type of injecting equipment do you use, e.g. gauge of needle, size of barrel, make of syringe?
- how often do you re-use your injecting equipment?
- do you know how syringe sharing can transmit HIV?
- do you consider yourself to be at risk?
- do you want to change your injecting/drug use in any way?
- which service is most appropriate to you?, e.g. syringe exchange, DDU, GP?
- do you ever borrow someone else's syringe – under what circumstances?
- do you lend your syringe to other users – under what circumstances?
- do you share syringes with your sexual partner(s)?
- do you know about your partner's syringe sharing?
- what syringe cleaning methods do you use – under what circumstances, i.e. for your own works; other people's works?
- what parts of your body do you inject into?
- how long does it take you to find a vein?
- do you alternate injection sites?
- do you clean injection sites? What with?
- are there physical problems as a result of injecting which require medical attention?
- what do you mix your drugs with, e.g. tap water, sterile water, citric acid (lemon juice)?
- how would you go about suggesting not sharing with partner or friends?

Modifying injecting techniques

Before HIV, injecting drug users were subject to a range of physical problems as a result of injecting unsterile drugs (drugs not designed for injection) and poor injecting techniques. In 1985, in a study of 119 clients attending St Mary's DDU, only one client cited AIDS as a reason for not sharing works – concern over Hepatitis B and general health were more common.[21]

The medical complications can involve:

- Hepatitis B (infection of the liver);
- abscesses – sterile due to irritant drugs or poor injecting technique; infected due to unsterile drugs and technique;
- septicaemia;
- sub-acute bacterial endocarditis – inflammation and damage to the lining of the heart caused by an infective organism, *Streptococcus viridans*);
- embolism – a substance such as air or impurities in illicit drugs carried by the bloodstream until it causes obstruction by blocking a blood vessel;
- thrombosis – narrowing of veins, causing blood clots;
- gangrene – due to damaged circulation and poor care of wounds;
- poor healing of wounds (due to inadequate general health and poor circulation);
- circulatory problems;
- scarring;

Good injecting technique is of considerable importance to the IDU's overall health. The following points are of particular importance:

(1) Advise the IDU to avoid sharing any injecting equipment including cookers, rinse water etc.
(2) Clean the injection site before injection. This can be done with soap and water or antibacterial swabs. The main value of antibacterial swabs is thought to be in the prevention of blood spillage following injection. Although a history of skin cleaning before injection has been found to decrease the risk of bacterial soft tissue infections and endocarditis.[22] Check that all air has been expelled from the syringe. Insert the needle, at a 45 degree angle, into the vein – the point of the needle should face the direction of the bloodflow. Once in the vein, withdraw the needle slightly to ensure it is properly in the vein; inject, then gently slide it out; swab again and apply gentle pressure.
(3) Avoid arterial points like the neck and groin. Arteries carry bright red blood; veins carry dark red blood. If users hit an artery the blood may also appear frothy or the plunger may be forced back by the pressure. Injecting into the artery will not have the desired

effect. If the IDU hits an artery they should remove the syringe, apply pressure to the site, raise the limb, and press down firmly for a minimum of 5 to 10 minutes. If still concerned, they should go straight to an Accident and Emergency Department. Injecting into arteries can lead to gangrene. If they are trying to find bigger veins these will be deeper under the skin surface; a bigger needle is thus required and, as these larger veins have more sluggish circulation, spasm is more likely to occur. If they are going to use veins with sluggish circulation – at the back of the knee, for example – then they should inject slowly. Arteries can be felt to pulsate only when they go over a bone; veins also pulsate but imperceptibly. The difference is that veins collapse when pressure is applied since they have less muscle in their walls.

(4) If the user does not alternate the injection site and persists in injecting drugs that are irritating to the tissues then the result is likely to be constriction of the veins (Fig. 3.1) and the formation of an abscess.[23] Veins have very little blood pressure so very mild damage can be sufficient to allow the sides to adhere if the vein collapses. If such an adhesion takes place it is likely to become permanent and the vein will disappear. Track marks are the result.

(5) Rotate injection sites. Many users spend a great deal of time looking for veins. Half an hour or longer is not unusual where the IDU has very poor peripheral circulation. They should try to use the superficial veins in forearms, the inside of elbows, hands and feet. But they should inject slowly in the veins of the hands and feet in order to avoid damage to fragile veins. Using a tourniquet will help identify veins that have not collapsed, providing it is not pulled too tight. Rubbing, tapping and clenching the fist first can also help. If the IDU is warm, then venous blood flow will be more obvious. They should inject with, not against, venous blood flow.

Good injection practice includes the following:

- try to develop ambidextrous injecting techniques;
- use new equipment whenever possible. (If you do not give out works yourself, then give them the addresses of needle and syringe exchanges and pharmacists who sell equipment.);
- avoid lending or borrowing injecting equipment. They may be more likely to lend the syringe if another IDU needs it;
- if they re-use their own equipment, mark it with an identifier in case it gets mixed up with someone else's;
- avoid bottled lemon juice and vinegar as a dissolving agent for

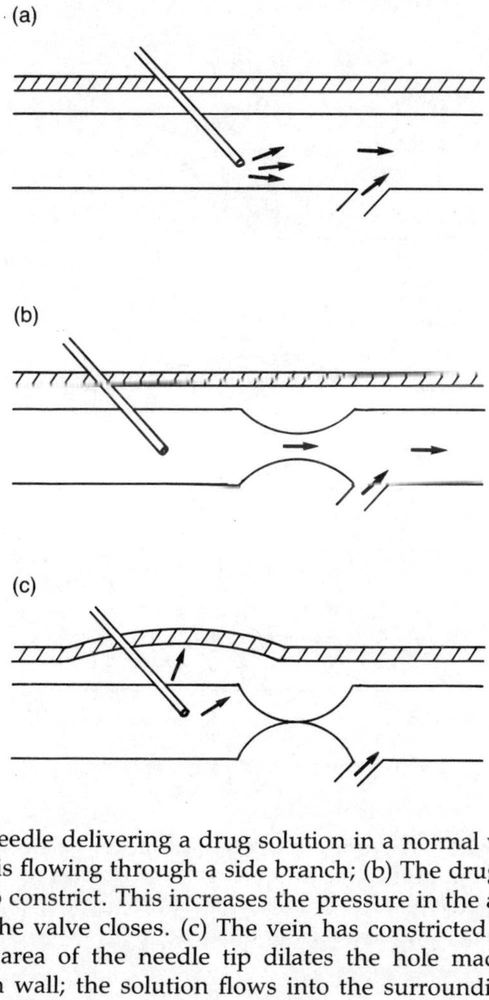

Fig. 3.1 (a) A needle delivering a drug solution in a normal vein. The valve is open and blood is flowing through a side branch; (b) The drug has irritated the vein causing it to constrict. This increases the pressure in the area of the needle and as a result the valve closes. (c) The vein has constricted totally. The high pressure in the area of the needle tip dilates the hole made by the needle through the vein wall; the solution flows into the surrounding tissue and an abscess is formed.[23]

heroin. The acidity will cause irritation to the injecting site; in addition, if bottled lemon juice is stale, certain microbes can grow in it. If possible, use sterile water when mixing their drugs;

- avoid injecting pharmaceutical drugs where fillers will act as an irritant. This includes Diconal, benzodiazepines and barbiturate powder.

In addition to infected abscesses caused by unsterile techniques, abscesses may also be caused by injecting drugs which are not meant

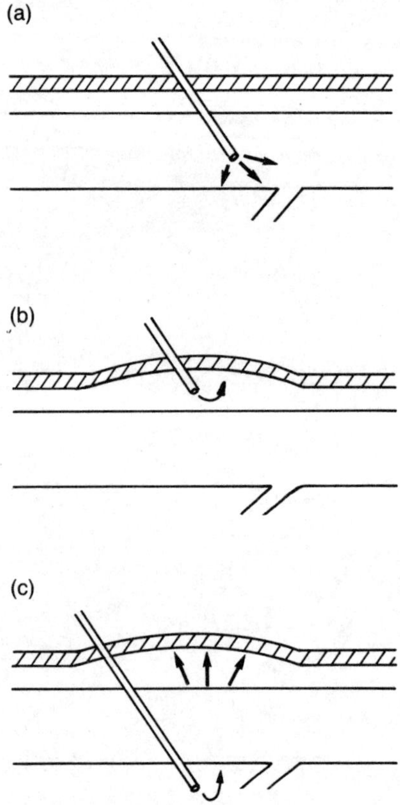

Fig. 3.2 (a) A needle delivering a drug solution into a normal vein; (b) The needle has pulled out of the vein and the solution is passing into the surrounding tissue; (c) The needle has penetrated the other wall of the vein so that the solution again passes into the surrounding tissue.

for intravenous use; they are the result of injecting ground up tablets such as Diconal, barbiturates, and tranquillizers.[24] Abscesses such as that shown in Fig. 3.2 occur where the vein has been missed. These unaffected abscesses may also be called sterile or cold. In addition, the skin over the injection site may slough off, leaving an ulcer.

If users inject into a muscle they should use area where there is plenty of muscle bulk the upper outer quadrant of the thigh muscle, for example, but they should also alternate these injection sites. If they 'skin pop', (i.e. inject sub-cutaneously) they should use forearms, thighs and stomach; this practice, however, carries a higher risk of developing an abscess.

Methods of syringe cleaning and disposal

Find out the disposal methods the client uses; some will bring their used works to a syringe exchange and this should be encouraged. If they can use a cinbin then so much the better. If they are not willing to do this and if the needle is detachable, advise them to take it off, (some IDUs bend or break it), put it into the barrel, insert the plunger, and then wrap it up well and bin it. Some needles do not detach from the barrel. In such cases clients have tended to re-sheath them or bend the needle. Whatever method they choose, the syringe should then be placed into an impermeable container and binned. Drink cans have been suggested as suitable containers. Some workers have voiced concern over this because of the trend to collect these cans for recycling. This highlights how necessary it is for the worker to establish what is most practical/realistic for the individual IDU in order that the client can undertake safe disposal to the best of their ability and is not overwhelmed by a list of do's and don'ts.

Before offering advice to a client, try cleaning some syringes and needles yourself first; it can be an extremely valuable learning experience. It will help elucidate the gap between information giving and carrying out these procedures in reality: you will become aware, for instance, of the amount of equipment, the time it takes, and the fact that the cleaning techniques will not be suitable for all syringes. Minor burns, needlestick injuries and spilt bleach are not uncommon occurences amongst drug workers given the opportunity to try out these cleaning techniques on training courses.

It is worth bearing in mind that disposable syringes are not produced with frequent re-use in mind. Whatever the cleaning method used, therefore, the quality of the syringe is likely to deteriorate fairly rapidly over time.

Disinfection fluids

Sodium hypochlorite (a common constituent of household bleach), gluteraldehyde, formalin, phenolics, ethyl and isopropyl alcohols, and strong acid, will all inactivate HIV at different concentrations.[25] There is no conclusive evidence on the most effective cleaning method for syringes. The current advice from the Expert Advisory Group on AIDS (UK) is as follows.

Washing up liquid method

(1) Put a generous squirt of washing up liquid in a cup and add cold water.
(2) Draw the liquid right up the needle and fill the syringe.
(3) Flush this away (not back into the cup).
(4) Draw up some more liquid and flush that away.
(5) Put some clean cold water in a container, draw it up into the needle and fill the syringe.
(6) Flush this away (not back into the clean water).
(7) Repeat stages 1 to 6 one or two more times.

Advantages
- uses substances that are readily available;
- liquid detergents have a demonstrated viricidal effect;
- quick procedure to undertake.

Disadvantages
- requires that the user has access to these substances and is in a situation where they can be used;
- the detergent/water solution needs to be sufficiently dilute to draw up into very thin gauge needles;
- the client needs to be advised against sharing rinsed water, and to ensure that the rinsed water is clean;
- it can sometimes be difficult to remove all the detergent from the syringe.

Bleach method

(1) Put some undiluted household bleach into a container.
(2) Draw this right up the needle and fill the syringe.
(3) Flush this away (not back into the bleach container).
(4) Repeat stage 3, above, once or twice more.
(5) Put some clean cold water in a container, draw this up into the needle and fill the syringe.
(6) Flush this away (not back into the clean water).

Advantages
- uses substances that are readily available;
- certain disinfecting agents have a demonstrated viricidal effect;
- a relatively quick procedure to follow.
- has been used with some success in outreach projects in the United States and in the UK.

Disadvantages

- bleach degenerates on exposure to light and heat; it also loses its strength over time;
- proprietary bleaches are usually sold in different strengths of solution;
- the use of this method may perish the rubber tip of the plunger, making it stiff to move; eventually bleach will corrode the needle;
- bleach can be inactivated by contact with organic materials such as blood, so it should never be re-used;
- the client needs to be advised to avoid sharing rinsed water, and to make sure that the rinsed water is clean;
- it has been suggested that bleach can harden blood plugs in the barrel of the syringe and therefore make them more difficult to flush out;
- thick bleaches will not draw up into thin gauge needles, such as 1 ml insulin syringes.

Boiling method

(1) Put some clean cold water in a container and draw this up into the syringe.
(2) Flush this away (not back into the clean water).
(3) Repeat stage 2 once or twice more.
(4) Take the syringe apart, i.e. if possible, separate plunger and needle from barrel.
(5) Put some water into a pan and bring to the boil.
(6) Put all the pieces of the syringe into the boiling water and leave for at least five minutes.
(7) Remove syringe pieces from boiling water (taking care not to burn yourself).

Advantages

- one of the most thorough cleaning methods.

Disadvantages

- requires access to a lot of equipment – saucepan and other containers, source of running water, cooker, source of energy;
- takes an average of 10–12 minutes from beginning to end (assuming a five-minute boil time) and access to all the necessary equipment at the start;
- may damage the rubber plunger, making it stiff to use;
- many makes of plastic syringes do not withstand boiling and dis-

tort or melt within five minutes, e.g. Sabre, all sizes; Sherwood–Monoject 1 ml, and S and N Everett 10 ml.

There has been much debate about the best cleaning methods to use. Obviously it is safest to use new equipment every time. However, the drug user may find themselves in a situation where new equipment is not available.

The most appropriate advice for each individual will depend on the following:

(1) The drugs the IDU injects and the size of the syringe they use. Many users still go to retail pharmacists for their syringes because of the wider choice of syringes and needles as well as their convenience and longer opening hours.
(2) The circumstances in which they might inject. What would be appropriate in a fully equipped kitchen will not be so in a public toilet or park.
(3) The cleaning methods the client has used in the past, if any.
(4) Whether the IDU is cleaning their own equipment for re-use or cleaning a borrowed syringe. They are more likely to use a more elaborate cleaning technique if using a borrowed syringe.

On the basis of this information, and in consultation with the IDU, an assessment of the feasibility and appropriateness of the various cleaning methods can be made.

Initiating behaviour change

Prior to the advent of HIV, the majority of research into behaviour change among drug users concerned assessment of their response to drug treatment regimes. Since HIV, more effort has gone into evaluating drug users' responsiveness to risk reduction information. Since much of the research is drawn from clinic/syringe exchange attenders, relatively little is known about the risk behaviours of drug users who are not in agency contact. Power *et al.*, in their comparison of an agency group and a group not in contact with drug agencies, found a significantly lower prevalence of injecting risk behaviours among the agency group.[26] Although more recent work carried out by this group suggests that non-attenders of syringe exchanges are also able to reduce their injecting risks.

If services are seen to be attractive then presumably more IDUs will want to use them. Services require resources in order to do this and many require significant policy alterations. User friendly services are often perceived to have a wider range of services available even if what they offer is equivalent to other more traditional units, i.e. they make a better job of selling their service.

Prescribing substitute drugs

Prescribing substitute drugs to opiate-dependent IDUs at the very least keeps them in contact with an agency that can monitor their state of health. Primary health care can be offered and essential health education carried out. Oral methadone is more likely to be considered here as the substitute drug because this drug dominates the debate on prescribing. The use of substitute drugs in the treatment of non-opiate dependence is practically non-existent. There is relatively little experimentation with alternatives of this sort, a fact that has significant implications for HIV prevention strategies. A large proportion of injectors will be non-opiate users.

There is concern that prescribing, when done on a maintenance basis, will inhibit positive change in the IDU and simply maintain the status quo. Prescribing also contributes to the 'silting up' of services and clients on maintenance may continue to inject street drugs anyway. These arguments may be valid but the reality for the user is long waiting times, elaborate and often inconsistent assessment procedures and often inflexible prescribing policies. According to Ghodse[27] most IDUs (85%) thought that stopping injecting could be easier if treatment were available more quickly. Few would argue with this.

Preliminary data both in Europe and the USA suggest that HIV seroprevalence is lower among clients who receive long-term methadone maintenance and who entered treatment before the onset of increasing seroprevalence within the local IDU population.

Prior to the advent of HIV, a number of studies have indicated that methadone maintenance produces significant improvements in levels of opioid use as well as in criminality and general health. Arguments against this have drawn criticism on these studies due to methodological flaws. Some studies have indicated little influence of treatment contact on overall outcome of drug use.[28] Well designed treatment comparison studies are rare; evaluation studies in the US indicate that length of time in treatment is an important predictor of treatment and post-treatment success, regardless of treatment modality.[29,30] One study found a relationship between length of time spent in treatment, decreased use of narcotics and other illicit drugs, and increased social productivity.[31] Dosage levels may also have an impact. In the United States programme, retention was improved by methadone doses of 50–100 mg, especially during the first six months.[32,33]

It is important to try and match the services to the client's needs. For clients with little evidence of psychopathology, it is likely that counselling and psychotherapy is no more effective than other ancillary services. It may be that what clients want is the choice as to whether or not they receive counselling. Preliminary studies suggest that low threshold clinics (where there is no commitment other than daily collection of medication) suggest utility and potential impact on reducing the spread of HIV infection.[34] A positive staff attitude and flexible treatment philosophy both positively influence patient retention.[35,36]

Regardless of educational level and addiction history, counsellors who have specific patient management skills significantly enhance patient retention and reduce intravenous drug use – in marked contrast to programmes with staff who lack these skills.[37,38] Having said this, it is difficult to maintain a positive attitude if you represent a service where the waiting list is so long that you spend the majority of your time turning people away. For some IDUs, being HIV positive at the very least means that they will have easier access to prescribing services, although as numbers increase this is by no means always the case. We now have enough knowledge to implement significant changes in prescribing, in drug treatment and HIV prevention. We could, in this author's opinion, make enormous headway if we put into practice what we already know.

Counselling and ancillary care

General practitioners

Many IDUs do not have a GP and many GPs are reluctant to take on IDUs because of their drug problem. Some GPs will agree to treat drug users, often in collaboration with a drug agency or community drug team who will advise the GP and provide counselling for the drug user. Since treatment places at DDUs and detoxification units are extremely limited, GPs are now playing an increasing role in treating drug users, a fact of some significance since one study estimated that GPs are seeing up to 44 000 new cases of opiate misuse a year.[24] Access depends first of all on whether or not the GP is willing to work with IDUs; this in turn means that the drug user either has to shop around or may obtain access through a drug agency. One survey of GPs in South London found a reluctance to care for IDUs, a lack of knowledge about AIDS, and an inability to offer counselling and advice on the subject.[39] Without support, many GPs who would otherwise be sympathetic to the idea of taking on drug users may feel unable to do so.

In discussing their own fears, one GP, a woman, mentioned her fear of doing house calls late at night to a drug-using couple. The GP surgery may therefore be more suitable for the stable long-term maintenance client who does not require counselling. The more chaotic user with special needs with be better served where support services are more concentrated at specialist drug agencies.

Outreach work

Many HIV prevention initiatives suggest that outreach work should form an important component in HIV prevention. However, what is less clear is what outreach work involves, how it should be done, and who is best fitted to carry it out. Outreach among drug users is not new it has already been carried out on a small scale since the late 1970s and early 1980s. Outreach services can provide the following:

- health education, risk-reduction counselling and support;
- provision of condoms, bleach and injecting paraphernalia, and, in some cases, health care;
- referral to drug services.

Some of the most encouraging examples of this approach are seen where outreach fits in with an overall concept of improved access to services. As an example of this, outreach workers in New Jersey offered discount tokens to IDUs which enabled them to get treatment at the local methadone clinic. Co-operative systems of this nature should be encouraged.

The issue of job satisfaction for the outreach worker is also a pertinent one: they often work alone; their colleagues may not have a clear understanding of the pressures of their job; there are particular environmental constraints to the work, and if their job consists of referring people for further treatment, there may be the frustrations of not seeing the work all the way through. Workers are often placed in situations of considerable personal risk and often work anti-social hours. There are few guidelines on how to do this work. Should they work alone or in pairs? What is the best approach to use with particular clients? What subjects do they need to cover? What characteristics should the outreach worker possess? Is a worker necessarily more effective if he or she is matched to the client's characteristics. If this means users and ex-users, the work may be putting them into situations where they are extremely vulnerable. What support services are required? Not surprisingly, the outreach workers who have had longevity in their career tend to have very individual working styles and good support systems. If outreach serves the function of encouraging IDUs to come into a service, then the service must accommodate this; there is no point, for example, in encouraging IDUs to get into treatment for their drug use if there are no treatment places available.

The matter of evaluation of service effectiveness can be particularly difficult. It is, however, essential if these services are to receive continued funding. The evaluation measures used need to be kept simple; you cannot necessarily do an hour-long interview with a client you meet on the street. The measures should be based on the objectives of the work itself, for example, education, which includes increased knowledge, support, behaviour change, uptake of syringes, condoms, etc.

One particular advantage of the community base is that the outreach worker will have a greater awareness of the local drug use conditions and be more sensitive to needs and changes in needs and will be able to identify new drug taking trends much more quickly than those working from less accessible services.

There are a wide range of settings for drug work. How each agency responds to HIV will depend on the context of the work, the resources available, and the motivation of the staff and the clients who use it. Each agency needs to decide how it will respond and what is appropriate and practical given these limitations. The possibilities include the following:

- prescribing services;
- provision of syringes, swabs, cinbins, tourniquets and sterile water. Flexible exchange policy;
- counselling and support;
- advice on welfare rights;
- syringe disposal facilities;
- afternoon or evening opening hours;
- medical care;
- family planning;
- well woman clinics;

- support/education groups;
- dietary advice and nutritional supplements;
- antenatal and maternity services;
- GP referrals and support;
- health education leaflets and other materials;
- telephone advice;
- residential facilities for drug users with AIDS;
- legal advice, prison visiting and liaison;
- supply of condoms, spermicides and dental dams;
- in-patient/residential detoxification;
- structured day programmes;
- HIV counselling and testing;
- outreach work;
- crisis intervention;
- skills/employment training;
- parenting skills; parent and toddler groups;
- housing advice and support;
- immunisation and screening;
- residential/out-patient rehabilitation;
- home delivery of injecting equipment (in rural areas);
- pharmacy liaison syringe exchange schemes;
- family work;
- mobile exchange and treatment units;
- automatic syringe dispensing machines.

Some HIV-related services do not require significant changes in agency policy; others do. HIV can have a significant impact both on the workload and on the unit's philosophy. It can serve to highlight broader improvements in the client's lifestyle but, conversely, it increases the challenge to the worker and can lead to confusion about his or her role. A practical working philosophy and clear objectives in assessment procedures can help to alleviate this. In order to achieve this, an accurate knowledge or evaluation of the needs of the local drug-using community is useful. The objectives of the service should be based on a combination of this information and a service philosophy (which should itself be acceptable to the workers). All of this will, of course, be influenced by financial constraints. Unfortunately, where drug work is concerned, financial constraints can be one of the greatest sources, of dissonance between what the IDU needs and what the service is able to provide.

References

1. Turner, C.F., Miller, H.G. & Moses, L.E. (1989) *AIDS: sexual behaviour and intravenous drug use*. New York: National Academy Press.
2. Anhalt, N.S. & Klein, M. (1976) Drug abuse in high school populations. *American Journal of Drug and Alcohol Abuse*, **3**, 589–603.
3. Brook, J.S., Whiteman, M. & Gordon, A.S. (1982) Qualitative and quantitative aspects of adolescent drug use: interplay of personality, family and peer correlates. *Psychological Reports*, **51**, 1151–63.
4. Sheehan, M., Oppenheimer, E. & Taylor, C. (1988) Who comes for treatment?: drug misusers at three London agencies. *British Journal of Addiction*, **83**, 311–20.
5. Kandel, D., Kessler, R. & Margulies, R. (1978) Adolescent initiation into stages of drug use: a developmental analysis. In *Longitudinal research on drug use: Empirical findings and methodological issues*. (Ed. D. Kandel.) Washington DC: Hemisphere Publishing Corporation.
6. Gold, M.S., Dackis, C.A., Pottash, A., Extein, I. & Washton, A. (1986) Cocaine update: from bench to bedside. *Advances in Alcohol and Substance Abuse*, **5**, 35–60.
7. Schuckit, M.A. (1984) *Drug and alcohol abuse: a clinical guide to diagnosis and treatment*. 2nd edn. New York: Plenum.
8. Gawin, F.H. & Ellinwood, E.H. (1988) Cocaine and other stimulants: actions, abuse and treatment. *New England Journal of Medicine*, **318**, 1173–82.
9. Dixon, J. (1990) HIV prevention in experimental and recreational drug users. *The Newsletter, The International Working Group on AIDS and Drug Use*, **5**, (1), 12–14.
10. Stall, R., McKusick, L., Wiley, J., Coates, T., *et al*. (1986) Alcohol and drug use during sexual activity and compliane with safe sex guidelines for AIDS: The AIDS Behavioural Research Project. *Health Education Quarterly*, **13**, 359–71.
11. *Drug misuse: a basic briefing* (1988). Central Office of Information. London: HMSO.
12. Waldorf, D. (1970) Life without heroin: some social adjustments during long term periods of voluntary abstention. *Social Problems*, **18**, 228–42.
13. Hanson, B., Beschner, G., Walters, J.M. & Bovelle, E. (1985) *Life without heroin*. Massachusetts: Lexington Books.
14. Klee, H., Faugier, J., Hayes, C., Boulton, T. & Morris, J. (1990) AIDS related risk behaviour: polydrug use and temazepam. *British Journal of Addiction*, **85**, (9), 1125–32.
15. Des Jarlais, D.C., Friedman, S.R. & Marmor, M. (1987) HTLV-III/LAV-associated disease progression and co-factors in a cohort of IV drug users. *AIDS*, **1**, 105–111.
16. Kaslow, R.A., Blackwelder, W.C., Ostrow, D.G. *et al*. (1989) No evidence for a role of alcohol or other psychoactive drugs in accelerating immunodeficiency in HIV-1 positive individuals. *JAMA*, **261**, 3424–9.
17. Stallard, A., Heather, N. & Johnson, B. (1987) AIDs and intravenous drug

use: what clinical psychology can offer. *Bulletin of the British Psychological Society*, **40**, 365–8.

18. Black, J.L., Dolan, M.P., De Ford, H.A., Rubenstein, J.A., Pen, W.E., Robinowitz, R. & Skinner, J.R. (1986) Sharing of needles among users of i.v. drugs. *New England Journal of Medicine*, **314**, 446–7.
19. Blattner, W., Biggar, R.J., Weiss, S.H., Melbye M. & Goedert, J.J. (1985) Epidemiology of human T-lymphotropic virus type III and the risk of acquired immunodeficiency syndrome. *Annals of Internal Medicine*, **103**, 665–70.
20. Donoghue, M.C., Stimson, G.V., Dolan, K. & Alldritt, L. (1989) Changes in HIV risk behaviour in clients of syringe exchange schemes in England and Scotland. *AIDS*, **3**, 267–72.
21. Mulleady, G., White, D., Phillips, K. & Cupitt, C. (1990) Reducing sexual transmission of HIV for injecting drug users: the challenge for counselling. *Counselling Psychology Quarterly*, **3**, (4), 325–41.
22. Herb, F., Watters, J.K., Case, P. & Pettiti, D. (1989) Endocarditis, subcutaneous abscesses and other bacterial infections in intravenous drug users and their association with skin-cleaning at drug injection sites. V International Conference on AIDS, Montreal (Abstract ThDO4).
23. Hecker, J. (1988) Improved techniques in i.v. therapy. *Nursing Times*, **84**, (34), 28–33.
24. Glanz, A. & Taylor, C. (1986) *Findings of a national survey of the role of GPs in the treatment of opiate misuse* (3 parts). British Medical Journal, **293**, 427–30.
25. Jeffries, D.J. (1988) Control of infection policies. In *The ABC of AIDS* (Ed. M.W. Adler.) London: *British Medical Journal*.
26. Power, R., Hartnoll, R. & Daviaud, E. (1988) Drug injection, AIDS and risk behaviour: potential for change and intervention strategies. *British Journal of Addiction*, **83**, 649–54.
27. Ghodse, A.H., Treganza, G. & Li, M. (1987) Effect of fear of AIDS on sharing of injecting equipment among drug abusers. *British Medical Journal*, **295**, 698–9.
28. Stimson, G.V., Oppenheimer, E. & Thorley, A. (1987) A seven year follow up of heroin addicts: drug use and outcome. *British Medical Journal*, **i**, 1190.
29. Simpson, D.D. (1979) The relation of time spent in drug abuse treatment to post-treatment outcome. *American Journal of Psychiatry*, **136**, 1449–53.
30. De Leon, G., Andrews, M.P.A., Wexler, H.K., Jaffe, J. & Rosenthal, M.S. (1979) Therapeutic community dropouts: criminal behaviour five years after treatment. *American Journal of Drug and Alcohol Abuse*, **6**, 253–71.
31. Simpson, D.D. (1981) Treatment for drug abuse: follow up outcomes and length of time spent. *Archives of General Psychiatry*, **38**, 875–80.
32. Garbutt, G.D. & Goldstein, A. (1972) Blind comparisons of three methadone maintenance dosages in 180 patients. In *Proceedings of the Fourth National Conference on Methadone Treatment*, New York, 411–14.
33. Dole, V.P., Nyswander, M.E. & Des Jarlais, D. (1982) Performance-based rating of methadone maintenance programmes. *New England Journal of Medicine*, **306**, 169–71.
34. Yancovitz, S., Des Jarlais, D., Peyser, N., *et al.* (1988) Innovative AIDS risk

reduction project: interim Methadone clinic. IV International Conference on AIDs, Stockholm.

35. Brown, B.S., Jansen, D.R. & Benn, G.J. (1975) Changes in attitude toward methadone. *Archives of General Psychiatry*, **32**, 214–18.
36. Anglin, D.M. & McGlothlin, W.H. (1984) Outcome of narcotic addict treatment in California. In *Drug Abuse Treatment Evaluation: Strategies, Progress and Prospects*. (Eds. F.M. Times & J.P. Ludford.) National Institute on Drug Abuse, Rockville, 106–28.
37. Aiken, L.S., Lo Sciuto, L.A., Aussetts, M.A. & Brown, B.A. (1984) Paraprofessional versus professional drug counselors: diverse routes to the same goal. *International Journal of Addiction*, **19**, 153–73.
38. Ball, J.C., Lange, W.R., Meyers, C.P. & Friedman, S.R. (1988) Reducing the risk of AIDS through methadone maintenance treatment. *Journal of Health and Social Behaviour*, **29**, 214–26.
39. Sibbald, B. & Freeling, P. (1988) AIDS and the future general practitioner. *Journal of the Royal College of General Practice*, **38**, 500–2.

Chapter 4

Pre-test Counselling

Introduction

The chemicals which our immune system produces in response to invasion by a foreign particle (or antigen) are called *antibodies*. These antibodies stick onto the surface of the antigen and stop it from working. We produce different antibodies in response to different antigens. Our immune systems produce antibodies in response to infection with the HIV virus. Unfortunately, these antibodies appear to be relatively ineffective in neutralising the virus.

HIV antibody test

As the name implies, the HIV antibody test detects the antibodies produced by the immune system in response to invasion with HIV. Usually people produce sufficient levels of antibody for detection within three months following infection with HIV. On rare occasions this may take longer. If someone is tested within this three-month period there is a strong likelihood of a false negative result.

A positive test result is not necessarily a diagnosis of AIDS. It means that the individual has come into contact with HIV, produced antibodies to it, and must therefore assume they are potentially infectious. A positive result does not tell you when or if you will develop AIDS. Nor does it tell you when you became infected. In the UK, antibody testing is undertaken by a method known as ELISA: a positive test result is double checked by using a different technique, usually Western Blot. A positive test result is thus usually very reliable.

A negative result should be interpreted in the light of the time lag between engaging in risk-taking behaviour and having the test. In cases where there is the possibility that the time lag was insufficient, it is sometimes recommended that the test be repeated after an interval of three to six months in order to be more certain about the validity of the result. The person is asked to refrain from engaging in risk activities for HIV in the intervening period. Depending on where the test is done and on the demand, it can take two to three weeks before the result is obtained.

The aims of pre-test counselling include the following:

- to ensure that the individual is fully informed and prepared for the implications of having a positive or negative result;
- to provide the individual with the necessary risk reduction advice regardless of the test result.

Other diagnostic tests

Virus culture

The HIV virus can be cultured in laboratory conditions from blood and some other body fluids. This is a complex, labour intensive and expensive procedure. It is therefore not generally undertaken unless people have immune deficiencies which are not attributable to HIV, or in babies born to seropositive mothers, to ascertain if transmission of HIV has occurred. The problem with a negative virus culture in such infants is that it may simply indicate that the virus has not been successfully grown. Most laboratories achieve something like a 60 to 80% success rate. One negative virus culture by itself therefore, is not considered sufficient to rule out the possibility of a positive diagnosis (see also Chapter 8).

Saliva testing

HIV antibodies can be found in low concentrations in saliva (approximately 1000 times less concentrated than in blood). The current test is about 99% efficient and is only used for epidemiological surveys into HIV prevalence, i.e. the results are not used for individual diagnosis.

Promising results have also been obtained in detecting HIV-1 antibody in urine, even although the virus is found to be approximately 10 000 times less concentrated than in blood. A non-invasive test for HIV would help relieve the undoubted distress experienced by many IDUs whose collapsed veins make taking blood an uncomfortable, and frequently painful, experience.

The effect of HIV testing on behaviour

More is known about the behavioural effects of testing on risk-taking behaviour among gay men than in any other group of individuals. Where studies on IDUs have taken place the results are ambiguous. In the US, Casadonte *et al.*,[1,2] found a reduction in risk taking among IDUs following testing. Those who tested positive reported greater risk reduction than those who tested negative. Overall, there was more change in injecting rather than in sexual behaviour. In another study[3] notification of test results to pregnant drug users was associated with increased use of crack in both seropositive and negative women.

According to one study carried out in Italy[4] knowledge of a positive result led to greater risk reduction than amongst negative or untested individuals. However, these workers also concluded that a negative result may give the drug user a 'false sense of security' and may contribute to the perpetuation of unsafe practices. In basic terms, not enough is known yet about the way drug users respond to testing. In work carried out at St Mary's, it was clear that many drug users felt that they were HIV antibody positive as a result of the risk practices that they had engaged in. However, they were reluctant to have their fears confirmed by having the test done. Uncertainty seemed to be the more acceptable psychological state, although, at the same time, many wanted to talk about it. Our own researcher, when interviewing IDUs, was struck by the number of clients who wanted reassurance from her that they had made the right decision not to have the test. Avoiding having one's worst fears confirmed is not an uncommon human reaction. Having the test done and then not going back for the result also occurs. Irrespective of testing, pre-test counselling on its own should not be underestimated as a vehicle for motivating change. On the other hand, testing is often appealing to the worker because it seems like 'something concrete' that can be done.

The worker's job is to provide the necessary information and risk reduction advice. Ultimately, whether or not to have the test is the client's decision, whatever views the worker holds. There is now probably more to offer the antibody-positive client in terms of prophylactic medication than there was a few years ago, although no cure can be offered. However, the enormous psychological and emotional impact of this test continue to remain.

Sometimes the worker's own opinion on whether testing is a good or bad thing will colour the way in which they present the pre-test information to the client. As has been said, the decision whether or not to have the test rests with the client; the worker should present the facts in as impartial a manner as possible whatever personal views they hold about whether testing is a good or bad thing.

In order for there to be benefits to the client from HIV testing, they need to have access to adequate pre-test counselling and post-test support. The opportunity for management of HIV infection also needs to be available to them as there seems to be growing support for the advantages of early detection both in treatment of opportunistic infections and for anti-viral therapies.

Testing may be considered in the following situations:

- before deciding to become pregnant or father a child and during pregnancy;
- in order to reduce uncertainty about HIV status;
- in order to consider drug interventions such as AZT;
- to support behavioural change;
- before embarking on a sexual relationship where the couple do not wish to practise safer sex.

The legal basis of confidentiality

Testing is available in a wide variety of settings, including STD clinics, drug units, syringe exchanges, ante-natal clinics and hospitals. The length of time you have to wait for a result and the extent of pre-test counselling will vary from setting to setting. It is useful to find out the policy on confidentiality where testing is carried out. Are results recorded in the client's notes? Who will be informed? Who will have access to these results? How is the information stored? There may be different standards of confidentiality and different legal implications regarding confidentiality depending on the setting where testing takes place. An STD or GUM clinic, for example, will be bound to comply with the Venereal Diseases Regulations (1974), limiting disclosure of patient information, except under specified circumstances. GPs and other hospital departments will not be bound by these regulations, although other confidentiality policies are likely to be in place.

Consent

It is not necessary in law for written consent to be given for the HIV antibody test to be carried out, but written evidence is important should a dispute arise. It can also act as a basic checklist that the necessary pre-test information has been covered.

Taking blood with consent but without knowledge of the reason for it being taken does not constitute battery, so blood may be taken for, say, ante-natal screening and then tested for HIV. Consent is not conditional on it being used for the stated purpose only. If you ask the doctor what your blood is going to be used for, you can insist that only named or agreed tests are carried out. In practice such questioning is a very difficult thing for people to do. Many of us are not used to asking our doctors for more information than we are provided with. In one situation a doctor was taking more blood from the patient than was necessary for the HIV test; the nurse working with her, although concerned about this, felt unable to ask the doctor what the rest of the blood was going to be used for. It is easy to say 'ask your doctor for more information'; it is much more difficult to do so in practice.

Pre-test assessment

It is important to establish the client's reason(s) for wanting to have the HIV antibody test – i.e. the risk activities engaged in and levels of risk. It is important to assess the client's level of understanding of what the test is, their knowledge of HIV and AIDS, its outcome and treatments. Most people expect (or hope) that the result will be negative. Exploration of the client's level of knowledge of HIV can enable the counsellor to move on to assess the client's support and coping resources should they turn out to have a positive result. Most people have great difficulty in exploring the personal consequences of a positive result. It is important to at least attempt to do this so that the client fully appreciates the implications of the test and both the worker and the client have some idea of how to proceed should the result be positive.

The content of pre-test counselling should cover the following areas:

- the limitations of the test – what it will and will not tell you;
- sexual and injecting risk reduction (Chapters 3 and 6);
- the practical implications of a positive result – insurance, mortgage, etc.;
- the impact that a positive result may have on the person's life;
- the medical management and treatment options available to the client, if any (bearing in mind that expensive drug therapies may not be universally available);
- how long the person will have to wait for the result and the standard procedure for giving results – i.e. not over the telephone.

Community health care when the result is positive

General practitioners

If the drug user has a GP who is involved in their medical care, then it is recommended that they tell that GP if they have a positive HIV antibody result. This is in order that the GP can participate fully in the client's care and take appropriate action if the client shows signs of HIV infection. The drug user may not want to do this and the issue should be fully discussed. If they are unhappy about the GP's involvement, they may wish to change to another GP; alternatively, they may opt for seeing the specialist at the local STD clinic. The disadvantage of this is that the STD clinic will not be available for emergency house calls. We have found that many clients without GPs will turn up at the hospital if they are feeling ill (some have tried, usually unsuccessfully, to call out ambulances).

It may be worth warning the client to ensure that any non-STD specialists they come into contact with at the hospital do not automatically inform their GP of their HIV status in the course of writing to them to report on the treatment they have received. If the client applies for life assurance, they will be asked by the insurance company to give the name(s) of any doctor(s) they have had for the past five years. Once they give their consent to the company to contact their doctor, the company will ask about risk-related activities, and HIV status. The client can ask to see the doctor's report before it is sent, but the doctor cannot withhold information. If the GP does the HIV antibody test and is also the doctor for the client's spouse, the GP may feel morally compelled to tell the spouse about a positive test result to protect their other patient, although it is their choice whether or not to do so. Legally, doctors are allowed to break confidentiality in such instances where another person's health is involved. In practice this is unlikely to happen without prior discussion with the HIV-positive partner.

Dentists

It is recommended that the drug user inform their dentist of a positive result in order that the dentist can take any precautions he/she feels necessary. In basic terms, however, dentists should employ adequate standards of infection control for all clients. Drug users frequently neglect their dental care; if they go to the dentist they often require fairly extensive treatment, not a particularly reinforcing scenario. It is useful to have the names of local dentists who will treat seropositive clients sympathetically, who are aware of IDUs' anxiety about pain control and are willing to consider higher levels of analgesia for these clients.

Police and the prison service

If the police discover a suspect's HIV status it is likely to go on their files and to be kept there. This may have several implications if a client is imprisoned, including, usually, the imposition of viral infectivity restrictions (VIR). This means segregation of HIV-positive inmates in separate units, withdrawal of association, and restriction of access to exercise and recreational facilities.

Life insurance, mortgages, employment and travel

Life insurance

Insurance may not be uppermost in the mind of the drug user at a time you see them, but it may become an issue in the future. If they apply for insurance there will probably be some questions on the application form which relate to HIV such as, 'Have you ever been refused as a blood donor?' 'Have you ever attended a venereal diseases clinic?' There will probably also be questions about drug and alcohol use. Clients can be refused on the grounds of previous history of drug abuse. Even with a negative antibody test result they may be refused – insurers are unlikely to give the reasons for this, nor are they required to do so. It helps to make general enquiries first rather than committing yourself and then being turned down since subsequent insurers may draw adverse inferences from previous refusals.

If the client lies about their status the contract will not be binding and the company can refuse to pay out in the event of a claim. Even if not asked for them, the client has a duty to reveal material facts. It is better not to have the test and apply for insurance, but again the company has the choice to refuse or accept. Some companies insist on a HIV test and negative result for some applicants, for example, in the case of two men who jointly apply for a mortgage. This is, of course, discriminatory, but not contrary to the Sex Discrimination Act since it can be scientifically proven that those with the virus have an increased risk of premature death and is therefore justified on actuarial grounds.[5]

Alternatively, the client may be offered insurance at a higher premium if the company thinks they are 'high risk'. Recently, the initiative to develop AIDS-exclusion policies has foundered. These provide life insurance cover excluding AIDS-related causes but these types of policy are not acceptable for mortgages.

Mortgages

Without life insurance there will be difficulties in obtaining a mortgage. Endowment mortgages, for example, require life assurance and will not be granted without it. Repayment mortgages on the other hand do not require life assurance but some lenders will insist that a mortgage protection policy is taken out. This pays off the mortgage should the holder die before the mortgage is fully paid up. Again this may not be a priority issue for drug users: if it is, however, there are certain mortgage arrangements that can get around the problem.

Employment

There have been cases where employers have discriminated against seropositive people and those associated with 'high risk' groups. GPs are often asked to provide information about a job applicant's health to prospective employers if the person signs a consent form when applying for the job.

The fact of being HIV-positive does not mean that you are less able to work than anyone else. There is no reason why present or prospective employers need to know. Advice to employers not to discriminate against employees on the basis of HIV status (circulated by the Department of Employment) is not legally binding and is also subject to individual interpretation. In some cases, discrimination has led to unfair dismissal or exclusion from certain jobs. Other employers have proved to be more reasonable – one large retail company, for example, referred an employee with AIDS for counselling to help him cope better with his work. They also complied with a request for his transfer to less strenuous work in another department.

Many drug users have no legal protection in the first place as a result of the 'off the cards' nature of a lot of the work that they are involved in. Some clients may decide to tell their employer when their work capacity is adversely affected by illness progression. Even then, HIV does not need to be the given cause should the client not wish to disclose this.

Travel

Many countries operate restrictions on the issue of visas and immigration on the basis of an individual's HIV status. Some countries will require proof of a negative result before they will issue a visa or work permit. Detailed advice on travel restrictions should be sought from the HIV and AIDS support agencies.

Tattoos

Many drug-using clients are tattooed, some professionally and some 'DIY'. People wishing to be tattooed should seek the services of a professional tattooist who has scrupulous standards of hygiene, i.e. uses new or sterile needles for each client. Similar precautions apply with ear piercing and electrolysis. With 'DIY' tattooing these are less likely to apply – often this type of tattooing is done by prison inmates, using unsterile equipment.

As a basic hygiene expedient, drug-users should also avoid sharing razors or toothbrushes.

As a matter of general policy, it is usually recommended that a client has time to consider the implications of the test before having blood taken, particularly in respect to the possibility of a positive result. There can be a lot of information to take in at one go and, in addition, all of this risk-reduction advice is relevant whether or not they decide to have the test.

References

1. Casadonte, P.P., Des Jarlais, D.C., Smith, T. *et al.* (1986) Psychological and behavioral impact of learning HTLV-III/LAV antibody test results. Presented at the Second International AIDS Conference, Paris, June 23–25.
2. Casadonte, P.P., Des Jarlais. D.C., Friedman, S. & Rotrosen, J. (1988) Psychological and behavioral impact of learning HIV test results in i.v. drug users. Presented at the Fourth International AIDS Conference, Stockholm, June 12–16.
3. Cancellieri, F.R., Holman, S., Sunderland, A., Fine, J., Bihari, D. & Landesman, S. (1988) Psychiatric and behavioral impact of HIV testing in pregnant drug users. Presented at the Fourth International AIDs Conference, Stockholm, June 12–16.
4. Sasse, H., Salmaso, S., Conti, S. & Rezza, G. (1988) Significance of HIV antibody testing as a preventative measure in intravenous drug users. *AIDS*, **2**, No. 5., 402–3.
5. Sex Discrimination Act (1975) section 45.

Chapter 5

Post-test Counselling

Introduction

The extent of post-test counselling may cover anything from a single visit by the client to receive an antibody test result, to in-depth long-term support to the client, their partner, family and friends. Drug workers are thus often well placed to offer such long-term support, since they may indeed see the client over a considerable period of time. The worker may already be aware of the lifestyle changes the client needs to make. The drug worker may not always be in the position of being the one to give test results to clients, but the client may come to them after they have been tested elsewhere, and want to talk about it. At the present time many drug workers find themselves in the position of counselling the client when they have had a negative result. The worker has to encourage the client to practise safer sex and safer drug use. It can be very difficult to get the client to recognise that these behaviour changes are still necessary.

In the aftermath of a positive result, the antibody-positive IDU may seek out the counsellor in order to find a shoulder to cry on or they may want to go over the 'facts' again in order to try to make sense of it for themselves. The chances are that if you bombard the client with information they will be unlikely to take it in; nor are they likely to appreciate it if, after coming to you for support, you overwhelm them with questions or a formal history taking. Give the client time for questions, check out their understanding, and be sensitive about striking an appropriate balance. It helps if you already have a relationship with the client. If you do know the client it is easier to put the information and advice into an appropriate context.

Breaking the news

If you are the person who has to give the client a positive test result, they are likely to be in shock whether or not they 'expected it'. Shock will limit their ability to take in information. Try to keep the messages clear and ask the client for feedback on what you have said to them. The lasting impact of this initial contact should not be underestimated. Do not feel you have to deliver all the news at once; wait for questions. Some clients report that they received little or no pre/post test counselling at this time. This may in fact have been the case, but it may also be the case that they were not in a condition to absorb the information as a result of shock, denial, or the influence of drugs. Much information will need to be repeated after the client has had time to take the result in.

There is no easy way to break bad news. Try not to be vague as avoidance of the facts can add to uncertainty and fear. We can give the client hope by emphasizing the options, but must not lie about these. Try to avoid issues of prognosis in terms of estimates of life expectancy and chances of developing AIDS. Tell the client what can be done about his or her condition, i.e. how further tests will give more information about their health, and the treatments they can choose to take (if indeed these are available).

As procedures for breaking the news of a positive test result, the following may be helpful:

- make sure you can be alone with the client and have the time to be with them;
- never give results over the telephone;
- try to avoid giving results on a Friday. The person may need support and be unable to obtain this over the weekend;
- provide lifelines – telephone numbers and contacts of support groups, syringe exchanges, STD clinics, etc.;
- provide written leaflets and information if this is appropriate, i.e. if the client can read and there is no danger that an 'inappropriate person' will come across this information;
- find out what the results mean to them and ensure that the person understands that a positive antibody test is not the same as having AIDS;
- go over the facts about the virus, particularly the routes of transmission;
- emphasise what not to worry about: i.e. casual contact; saliva; the fact that the virus is not airborne and cannot be caught from shared household equipment, toilets and other facilities;
- advise them not to share anything likely to be contaminated with blood, e.g. razors, toothbrushes. In the case of blood spillages, a solution of one-part bleach to ten-parts water is sufficient to clean it up;

- advise the client not to donate blood, organs, or semen and if they carry an organ donor card to destroy it;
- go over sexual and injecting risk-reduction advice;
- find out about the drug user's practical needs like welfare, grants, housing situation. How can you help with this?

Finally, offer an appointment within seven days. If you do not operate an appointment system let the client know the times they can drop in to see you. At this stage it helps if you can be flexible.

Some clients will have the test, but not go back for the result; alternatively, if they do go back, they do not want to be told the result. This situation can be very difficult for the worker who is faced with a dilemma. They may know that their client's result is positive, but cannot tell them. The burden that this can place on the worker should not be underestimated. The likelihood of this situation arising is reduced if the client can be shown that support and medical care are available. This is where having a good policy of health care for all clients makes sense so that even if the HIV-positive client is not getting prophylactic medication, they can at least have regular check-ups and opportunistic infections can be treated quickly. This can go a long way towards reassuring the client that they could receive the test result and be able to cope.

With drug use and HIV we often have to work with clients who come to services only when they are in crisis. As a result of this, there is little time for planning. The service is reactive and workers may feel under pressure. It also means that the client may not receive the most appropriate care at the time they choose to present in crisis. This is a fact of life in drug work. If the agency is set up to provide as many services as possible, as quickly as possible, then we have an ideal situation. However, most services are designed around a regular working day, not unreasonably, for the convenience of the workers. Greater flexibility in opening hours and service provision, and an accommodation of the client's priorities, will enhance the effectiveness and efficiency of care to the drug user. But, obviously, this requires a high level of resources, particularly with regard to extra staffing. Staff should never attempt to stretch themselves too thinly, for example, by attempting to provide 24-hour cover without adequate staffing levels and back-up.

Telling others the result

Initially it is advisable for the client to give themselves time to come to terms with the result before they tell anyone else. They will have had a chance to get over their own shock and be better informed; they will also be better able to cope with the reactions of others if they are not in a highly emotional state. I have encountered a number of clients whose response to being told they are HIV seropositive has been to go out and get stoned, and, as a result of this, blurt their result out to a number of people whom ordinarily they would not dream of telling. One client wondered if the staff of the DDU had told clients attending the clinic of his positive result, since, whenever clients met him they asked him if he had AIDS – he could not remember who he had told when he was stoned, but he had been heard to announce his result in the crowded DDU waiting room. It is best to warn clients about this possibility.

If you have the opportunity then discuss who they want to tell and how they will go about this. What will they say? What situation do they want to be in when they tell? What other information do they want to provide? What kinds of reactions will they have to cope with from others and from themselves? The worker can help by role playing this with the client and then exchanging roles. If the client remembers how they were given their own result, can they remember what was good or bad about how they were told? What tips could they pick up from this? How might they do it differently? If you see other members of the client's family or their partner, find out from the client what you can/cannot say to them. The client may want you to assist them in telling others and may bring their partner/relatives to see you. Again, negotiate with the client about what you can/cannot say to them.

For example, a client, 'Dave', was found to be HIV-antibody-positive. He had recently met a woman with whom he had started living. She was from Italy and her English was not very good. Initially he did not want to tell his girlfriend he was HIV-positive. He did not know how she would react and he was afraid she would leave him. His girlfriend was not a client of the DDU and Dave did not want her to come to the clinic (although she knew about his drug use). He was willing to consider condom use. He did not use them because his girlfriend was on the pill. Firstly, we discussed the different types of condoms and spermicides, and how to use them. One of the biggest stumbling blocks for this client was the way in which HIV had been associated with condom use – that it was tantamount to an admission of being

HIV-positive. We went through a number of explanations that he could use to account for his sudden desire to use a condom:

'You've been on the pill for a while and I'm worried about how this might affect your health.'

'I read an article recently that condoms help to prevent cervical cancer.'

'I'd like to take responsibility for the contraception for a change.'

'I've just had a talk with my drug worker about HIV. I don't want to have the test done, just yet; I don't have to as long as we use condoms.'

He decided on the final option. We discussed how and when he would introduce this to his partner, in what situation and the possible reactions she would have. Role playing involved practising different ways of saying it and swopping roles in order for him to have some idea of how these statements would sound to his partner, in other words, the practice of communication skills. Where condom use was concerned, we talked about how this might interfere with sex and how to cope with this initial awkwardness. Fortunately, his girlfriend reacted favourably to his suggestion to use a condom and stopped using the pill as a result of concerns she had about hormonal methods of birth control.

Obviously, this was not an ideal situation, but the client had set the goals and at the time was satisfied with what he had achieved. About four weeks later he told his partner he was HIV-positive; they remained together.

Agency responses

On receipt of a positive diagnosis, each individual will react differently with respect to their drug use. They may undergo a period of chaotic drug use and get completely obliterated so that they do not have to think about it. If this happens it tends to last a few weeks or months and then evens out again, although, in all cases, fluctuations will occur. Some people use a positive result as the spur for coming off drugs and making the most of their lives and stop or detoxify as a result. They may wish to continue injecting drug use and want prescribed injectables (however, they are unlikely to get these on the

NHS). They may want to get on a prescription for methadone in order to give themselves a break from street drugs, but without the serious intention of sticking to their prescription. Some clients express the anxiety that they are concerned about coming off drugs as this is inevitably a stressful experience and they are worried that stress may precipitate the development of illness. Some use this as a reason for not wanting to come off. Many residential treatment units have modified their programmes to reduce the stress associated with rehabilitation. This is a complex but important issue that many residential units have attempted to address.

If asked, many IDUs express the ultimate intention of coming off drugs at some time in the future. HIV can function as the crisis that precipitates coming off – particularly as it often coincides with increased access to support services. But with others HIV may increase pessimism and the feeling that there is no longer any point in coming off.

Whatever the individuals reaction, a range of prescribing, treatment and rehabilitation options should be available to all drug users who want them. In reality, this is not the case. One response to HIV infection and AIDS has been to prescribe very heavily to clients, John, for example, was a very verbally aggressive HIV-positive client with no symptoms. He had been to a number of different agencies. At his present agency he was being prescribed such an extensive cocktail of drugs that it was surprising he could still walk. There did not appear to be a clear rationale for this, other than keeping him quiet. Some may argue, what does it matter what drugs they are prescribed? Others strongly challenge this argument as being akin to giving up on the client. We need to be clear in our own minds where we stand on this issue and the reasons why we take up that position. Is prescribing in the best interests of the client or an expression (sometimes unconscious) of our own therapeutic pessimism?

It is important that we should not develop one aspect of drug services to the detriment of others. What is required is a comprehensive range of options. These options are still few and far between. A balance is therefore necessary between abstinence-orientated treatment and HIV prevention.

Basic medical care

Medical referral can be made at this time if the client wants it. The STD clinic at St Mary's Hospital is two minutes walk away from the DDU. However, on initial referral to the STD clinic for medical care, many clients manage to avoid getting there. Clients are often fearful that the doctor is going to tell them bad news, particularly if they have not had much medical care up until then. Avoidance of appointments can be one result of this, even though the client keeps requesting that further appointments be made. This has sometimes led to the client becoming quite ill before they will see a doctor. If possible, it can be helpful for the client to be accompanied to their first medical appointment.

Needless to say, the attitude of the medical and nursing staff has an enormous impact on whether clients will come back. If the client gets attached to a particular doctor, it can then be very unsettling for them if the medical staff change regularly – an occurence that is more likely among junior medical staff. This factor may have an impact on their compliance and willingness to attend. It goes without saying that the staff who have made the effort to inform themselves about drug issues and their clients' lifestyles are inevitably the most popular, as they tend to be more realistic about what changes are practical – it is not, for example, particularly helpful to tell the client at their first appointment that they should immediately stop smoking and taking drugs; but this has happened to a few clients and has been pretty effective at alienating them.

For drug users who have generally ignored and neglected their health, this sudden awareness of their physical health can be an unnerving experience for them and they can very easily overreact to symptoms. It is helpful if you can put their symptoms into an appropriate perspective. One client came to see me worried about memory problems and not being able to concentrate. He wondered if this meant he was developing dementia, 'I can hardly remember anything that happened over the weekend'. However, on further question, the client turned out to have had a rather generous intake of barbiturates, alcohol and Temazepam which may have had a slightly adverse effect on his recall! Hypochondriasis is not an uncommon reaction to a positive antibody test.

There is no way that colds and flu can be avoided but, depending on the baseline health of the client, they are not usually a problem. Heroin use suppresses the cough reflex; therefore, clients may not be aware of chest infections until they are well established. Clients may also be more susceptible to infections since the cough reflex to clear the lungs is also suppressed, thus leading to a build-up of mucus, etc. Many clients use Ventolin (salbutamol) inhalers. Although it is not clear which is the case, either there is a very high incidence of asthma amongst heroin users or they are self-medicating in order to alleviate the adverse effect of heroin on their breathing.

After a positive result, it will be necessary to discuss the symptoms and signs of HIV and AIDS with the client. This can be a very difficult issue as symptoms of anxiety and drug effects can mimic HIV-related disease. Raised anxiety about the appearance of symptoms can sometimes result in the client panicking at the slightest ailment. Occasionally, clients can become preoccupied with checking themselves for symptoms. Basically they should be told that they need to seek prompt treatment for chest complaints and other persistent infections.

The avoidance of adjunctive infection

Sexually transmitted diseases acquired after HIV infection have been implicated as co-factors for disease progression; routine screening for sexually transmitted diseases should therefore be built into medical check-ups. According to Cushman *et al.*,[1] injecting drug use in itself may result in immunological abnormalities such as false positive serological tests for syphilis. This makes it difficult to interpret syphilis results for HIV positive IDUs.[2]

Basic health care, hygiene and nutrition

The added importance of taking care of themselves, after an HIV-positive result, needs to be put into the context of the drug user's lifestyle. All aspects of the client's lifestyle should be discussed.

Nutrition

Drug users frequently report quite appallingly inadequate nutrition. Opiate use affects the digestion and the muscles controlling the digestive tract slow down. As a result, food remains in the gut for longer. This reduces the appetite and results in constipation. The preference for sweet foods, which provide bursts of energy, can contribute to this problem. Many clients seem to exist on sugary coffee and biscuits and report that they have no appetite for 'healthy food'. They often feel uncomfortably full as a result of eating 'a proper meal'. The drugs they use can suppress appetite and food does not tend to be a priority. Chemotherapy can produce further reductions in appetite. Under these circumstances it is a trifle unrealistic to expect them to suddenly adopt a health-conscious eating plan. It is first necessary to find out if they have money for food. If so, do they buy much food with it? Do they have cooking facilities? Secondly, do they have cooking utensils? If not, are there any charitable or support organisations willing to help out? If the drug user does not have cooking facilities, what money does he/she have to pay for food? What foods are they likely to choose? If the client has access to cooking facilities, it may be worthwhile suggesting easy-to-prepare nutritious foods, canned goods, packet soups or, if they can afford them, boil-in-the-bag meals.

If the drug user is a competent cook, make sure that they are aware of adequate kitchen hygiene, that they defrost food properly and ensure that it is thoroughly cooked.

Ask the client specifically what they eat, what they think a 'proper' meal is and what do they mean by the expression 'regular' meals. Eating more 'regular' meals is often reported by clients once they commence an oral methadone prescription. Nutritional problems can be complicated by pre-existing dietary disorders. Many clients seem to have abnormal eating habits, like binge eating, that predates their drug problem. As a result of HIV some 'fad' diets have been introduced; sometimes these can do more harm than good – the zen macrobiotic diet, for example, has been associated with some forms of malnutrition.[3]

Clients sometimes start to take vitamins rather than regular food intake. One client felt she had taken adequate care of her diet when she took her vitamins, plus two bottles of 'Thunderbird' a day and 'as much spirits as she could get her hands on'. It is often necessary to explain the importance of a good basic diet, before resorting to vitamin supplements which can be expensive. Unrelenting weight loss is a poor prognostic indicator for a person with AIDS.

Clients, however, may be losing weight, not as a result of HIV-wasting syndrome, but as a result of not eating. In some cases the provision of nutritional supplements such as 'Ensure' is a practical way of ensuring that the user gets their basic nutritional requirements. Some units have access to a dietitian and distribute dietary supplement drinks to those who need them. These can be very popular, so much so that their distribution requires considerable restraint on the part of the workers to limit them to those who need them as a result of AIDS or nutritional deprivation as opposed to those who want them because of the 'status' or because they cannot be bothered to eat. If these supplements are to be used appropriately, weight needs to be monitored on a regular basis. Some units with day care facilities offer the opportunity to prepare and eat food on the premises; others distribute free food from supermarkets that cannot be sold because it has just passed its 'sell by' date.

General hygiene

Precautions with regard to tattooing, acupuncture, etc., have already been mentioned in the pre-counselling section (Chapter 4). If the client has access to hot water and a sink then it is worth mentioning the importance of cleaning crockery and cutlery properly (i.e. using hot water and washing up liquid). It is also important to clear up blood and body fluid spillages with bleach and water and not to use bleach on the skin. One recently diagnosed HIV-positive IDU was found to have injected bleach because he had heard that it killed the virus.

Exercise

Exercise has been associated with improvements in immune system functioning.[3] Some sort of regular exercise is recommended. Some clients take to activities like cycling. One client bought a bicycle with his mobility allowance! The majority at least manage a daily walk to the chemist to pick up their methadone. Those who have taken up regular exercise, such as weight training, have mainly done so while in prison (that is, if they have been allowed to leave their cells).

Sleep

Sleep deprivation has also been associated with decreased immune system functioning.[4] As a result of their lifestyle, drug users often have very disrupted sleep patterns, frequently staying awake until the early hours and sleeping in until later in the day. It is very difficult to break this habit, especially if clients are still scoring street drugs. Prescribed methadone can help stabilise the user's lifestyle sufficiently to establish a more 'normal' schedule. However, those with regular employment or who have children, seem to be more likely to have regulated sleep patterns. Night sedation is not a long-term solution to the problem, but many clients seem to be much more likely to want a chemical answer to the problem than to actively attempt to re-establish a different sleep routine.

Many clients come to rely heavily on night sedatives such as Temazepam. Many of the sedative drugs routinely prescribed on hospital wards are habit forming, and may previously have been abused by the client. Some drug workers would question the advisability of continued prescribing on an outpatient basis as this may contribute to the IDU's drug problem. Whatever opinion you hold, it is clearly necessary for prescribing to be co-ordinated between the different agencies involved with the client. If the client is prepared to consider them, encourage the use of practical measures to improve sleep: regulated waking and sleep times; avoidance of stimilant drugs and heavy meals just prior to bedtime; milky drinks, relaxation methods and no exercise before bedtime; not going to bed until sleepy; avoidance of external noise and lowering lights.

Immunisation

Hepatitis B infection was common among IDUs prior to HIV and still is. It is useful to provide Hepatitis B vaccine for both the IDU and health care workers. This will help reduce further transmission to client contacts and reduce the risk from occupational exposure. It is advisable to seek professional guidance where the use of attenuated vaccine is required for immunisation for foreign travel.

Smoking and drinking

Cigarette smoking has been associated with decreased T4 cell counts.[4] Many IDUs smoke cigarettes; it is my experience that most of them feel they have enough constraints put on them by HIV without having to give up smoking as well. They might consider changing to a brand with lower tar levels or reducing their daily consumption. Similarly, with alcohol, although the evidence is less clear, alcohol may have an adverse effect on the immune system. Many IDUs increase alcohol consumption as their methodone script decreases.

Psychological and emotional reactions to HIV and AIDS

Stress and anxiety

There is evidence for the detrimental effect of stress on our immune functioning.[5] Taking drugs is one, maladaptive, way of coping with stress, but a better adjustment may be provided by adaptive coping methods, provided that these can be accommodated to the drug user's lifestyle. This is a problematic area because many drug users are used to taking the short cut to stress reduction and are unwilling to persevere with the practice necessary to master alternative coping techniques, such as relaxation training. In addition, being an illegal drug user constitutes a fairly high stress existence. There are also possible secondary gains: some users, for instance, will enjoy the excitement that comes from being outside the Law. Lower socio-economic status has also been shown to adversely affect susceptibility to stress-related illnesses. Increased illicit drug use as a response to a positive result is not an uncommon reaction. But if the client's drug use has been stable before diagnosis, it usually re-stabilises after a few weeks although this stability can be disrupted by subsequent stressful life events.

It may help both to brainstorm coping options with clients that would fit into their lifestyle and to provide training in alternative techniques. Many such techniques exist – cognitive therapy, biofeedback, yoga, etc. It is important not to underestimate the benefit of social support in improving the client's coping with stress. Not only talking it through with the worker, but being able to tell others and gain their support, can help enormously in reducing the client's anxiety. The overlap between anxiety, the effects of drug withdrawals, and some of the symptoms of HIV, can be alarming to clients (Fig. 5.1). These complicate accurate diagnosis, a fact which should be pointed out to them. There have been occasions when the client blames their HIV-related symptoms on their drug use since this is a more acceptable explanation than their physical deterioration.

Avoidance

Many clients who opt not to take an HIV test express the view that they think they are probably HIV-positive as a result of the behaviour they have engaged in but do not want this confirmed. Many will agonise over this decision and ask the worker for advice and reassurance that they have made the right one. This is not an unreasonable

Anxiety & Stress Related	*HIV & AIDS Related*	*Drug Related*
Headache	Toxoplasmosis, lymphoma, meningitis, encephalopathy	Bad hit, seisure due to barbiturate withdrawal
Skin conditions	Dermititis, folliculitis, dry skin as result of night sweats	Picking of skin due to cocaine use, abscesses, irritant drugs
Poor sleep	As result of raised temperature	Due to amphetamine & cocaine use
Heart disease	Direct effect of HIV, CMV infection	Sub-bacterial endo-carditis
Appetite loss	Candidiasis, CMV stomitis Drug treatment side effects	As result of heroin, cocaine use
Indigestion, ulcers	Cryptosporidium and other gut infections	Nausea, vomiting due to heroin, benzodiazepine withdrawals
Sweating	Night sweats due to seroconversion	Heroin withdrawals
Sexual problems	loss of libido, neurological problems	Due to heroin use
Leg aches	Muscle wasting caused by AZT, central and peripheral neuropathy	Damage to tissue as a result of injecting, abscesses, heroin withdrawals
Poor circulation	KS lesions, oedema	Calloused veins as result of repeated injection, poor injecting technique

Fig. 5.1 Symptom overlap examples.

reaction provided the IDU is prepared to consider any lifestyle changes they may need to make in order to reduce transmission risks and that they are clear that they do not want prophylactic treatments. The test, then, is not routine, nor is coping with a positive result.

Anger

The drug user may be angry at a number of things: at themselves for getting infected; the person who gave them the result; the worker who did not give them the drug treatment or syringes they wanted; their loss of freedom; their perception of a gloomy future; the person they think they acquired the infection from; the people they know who have taken the same risks and 'got away with it'. One client went back to his GP and accused him of causing the problem since he refused to give him a clean syringe when he needed one. Workers should not be surprised at having to cope with their clients' anger – they may be the only 'safe' person to express anger towards. One client went to another drug agency and accused a worker from the first agency of laughing at him when giving him his positive result; in fact the worker had provided appropriate and sensitive support. Anger can be one of the more difficult reactions to cope with, but anger not expressed can turn inwards and lead to depression. So, within limits acceptable to the staff, it should be safe for the client to express their anger. It is often an early reaction to diagnosis and can re-emerge at crisis points in the course of the illness.

Fear

The client may be fearful of death – most clients will be young people who have little or no prior experience of death. The same may be true for the worker. Fear of pain is common. In the early stages, when they begin to show symptoms, they may avoid going to see their doctor in case their worst fears are confirmed. Fear for their children – who will care for them? Fear of not being given sufficient pain control medication when illness is more advanced. Much is unknown, but a lot of fear can be alleviated beforehand by the giving of information, accurate feedback, and reassurance in order to minimise uncertainty, especially with regard to medical treatment.

Denial and disbelief

If a person has no symptoms it can be difficult to grasp the significance of the diagnosis. Since there is no physical manifestation of their condition they can push the issue to the back of their mind. This is a legitimate coping mechanism which is often seen in IDUs. Denial will affect the drug user's willingness to discuss HIV and related issues. Such discussion cannot, and should not, be forced on them. However, it does mean that the drug user may not have had the opportunity to work through their feelings before they become ill. As a result, there may be many unresolved conflicts at the time of their deaths which they may not have the time (nor the inclination) to talk about. This can mean that the experience is unnecessarily negative for the client; it can also leave the worker with unresolved feelings. It can also have implications for the drug user's family who may not have been involved at any stage prior to the drug user's death. However, the therapeutic goals are set by the client and not by us.

Even when symptoms are overt, the denial process can still operate. I visited an in-patient with TB and toxoplasmosis and all he talked about was getting out of 'this dump' and going back to Amsterdam to deal cannabis. He died four days later. As long as medical care is not compromised as a result, is it appropriate to get people to face up to their denial when they find it distressing to do so? They may never 'work through' all or any of the painful issues in their lives. Whose interests are served when we consciously stir up these issues in our clients?

It should be remembered that the drug user sets the pace and will talk when they want to and if we allow them to, but it may be the case that this never happens. Our clients are well defended emotionally by their drug use, but are in many other ways extremely vulnerable – that is why they go to the lengths they do in order to avoid looking at their problems.

Many clients are unused to talking about how they feel and may never have done so before. I am reminded of a woman client who turned up at the drug clinic just after she had received treatment for a serious outbreak of genital warts. She came into my office, sat down, and started to cry. She said that she did not want to talk about it and did not know what was wrong. As soon as she stopped crying, she got up and left. She had expressed her pain in the only way she knew how. As counsellors we may have expectations that the client will be able to verbalise their problems and feelings; this will not always be the case. This is not to say that counselling always has to be non-directive, especially where practical needs are concerned, attendance for medical check-ups, for example. It is often necessary for the worker to persist in 'nudging' the client to achieve the goals they have set for themselves.

Sometimes the user will disbelieve a positive result in the absence of symptoms on the grounds that the test was probably inaccurate and that they have friends who they have shared with and who have tested negative. One woman, tested without consent in hospital, became convinced that the positive result was wrong, but will not have this verified by a second test. In another case a client went on to the ward for pentamidine treatment and saw some of the people with AIDS who were there, and asked for a repeat HIV-antibody test. If clients come into contact with people in the more advanced stages of illness they will often ask for a repeat test because the possible significance of their diagnosis is brought home to them. However, others have found it very helpful to talk to people with AIDS who are more seriously ill than themselves and to find out how they have coped.

Self esteem

Low self esteem is a perennial problem for drug users. HIV has only added to this. The effect of low self esteem can lead the drug user to negate or diminish any positive actions or progress they may make. They must continuously be reminded of and reinforced for any positive action, however small.

Low self esteem can lead to terrible feelings of isolation. John, for example, goes down to the pub on Saturday nights to see his friends who are all non-drug users; none of them know about his HIV status and if they did he feels that they 'wouldn't come near me'. He feels he has to distance himself from his friends and 'keep up a front'. This gets particularly bad when they talk about AIDS when he is around. John's vulnerability contributes to his feelings of low self esteem.

Guilt

Clients may feel guilty about the people they have shared syringes with in the past, together with the possibility (or the reality) that they have infected their sexual partner and others. There may be guilt over loss of children through AIDS, infection in children, or the thought of leaving their children behind; guilt over the perceived waste of their lives.

Fatalism

I have seen this reaction to a positive HIV antibody test in a number of drug-using women who have IDUs as their sexual partners. Their overt reaction is 'well I expected it anyway' and not much else. The instinct for self preservation is low. This lack of concern for their own health can persist even where there is concern for the health of their partner or children.

Psychological, sexual and emotional problems

Sexual problems

Sexual problems may be long-standing and involve more than lack of interest in sex. Problems such as impotence, anorgasmia, and delayed ejaculation are common. Both partners need to be highly motivated to attend for sex therapy and often other difficulties in their lives seem more important. When asked about sexual difficulties in their lives a number of women mentioned 'passivity' (as they called it) in their sexual relationships – having sex when they did not really want it. Sexual problems may be more evident if the partner is a non-drug user. Drug use is a major cause of sexual problems – HIV can often exacerbate this situation. If both partners are motivated to seek help for this, then traditional sex therapy methods can be helpful.

Loss of control

The drug user may need to see a whole range of specialists, particularly when they become more severely immunocompromised. This can cause major disruptions in their lifestyle. There may be significant demands on their time: if they are not on a prescription they will have to obtain money for drugs; if they do not have a legitimate source of income they may have to commit crimes in order to raise the necessary cash and then spend time scoring drugs. If they have children they will only be free to attend appointments at certain times of the day. If their children are not at school, they will have to bring them along. Spending hours on end seeing different specialists, and undergoing different tests, may lead them to feel even more out of control of their situation. There may be anxiety about going into hospital and being unable to use the drugs they are using on the street.

It is useful to emphasise areas of their life where they do have control and to encourage them to build on these. Our clients consistently set themselves up to fail by picking tasks that are too much for them to cope with. It can help enormously to get them to break down their problems into achievable chunks and take on each one systematically. This is a problem-solving approach which can be either implicit in the way you work, or made explicit – i.e. worked out with the client using a problem solving grid similar to that used in assessment (Chapter 4).

We can facilitate the client's gaining control by avoiding over-helping behaviour. If there are things that the client can do for themselves, encourage them; otherwise you will increase the tendency to dump problems on you and you also prevent the client from learning to use their own resources. If a client has a problem which they can solve, then let them. Co-ordinated appointments can be a major help to cut down time spent waiting for treatment at hospitals. Explanations of treatment regimes and procedures, drug side effects, and the like, all provide the client with more information of what is happening to them and therefore more control. The relationship between control and prescribing substitute medication is interesting. At worst this will be entirely outside the client's influence; at best it will be a compromise negotiated between client and worker.

Depression and sadness

There are different kinds of depression – reactive, chronic and psychotic. The most common reaction to a positive HIV result is reactive depression – a normal reaction to loss, adverse circumstances, helplessness in changing the situation, and how much effort any change requires. Depression may occur periodically in response to events which remind the person of their positive status. It may also be a symptom of HIV-related dementia. Depression is characterised by a withdrawal from previously rewarding activities.

It is sometimes made manifest by an increase, *or* a reduction in interest in, and intake of, alcohol or illegal drugs. Chronic depression can be very difficult to diagnose accurately in people who take drugs. If the client's behaviour has always been influenced by drugs, it takes time to get to know the client before you can begin to distinguish normal behaviour from symptoms of depression; obviously moods will fluctuate anyway, but drug effects may mask symptoms which can be quite serious by the time the worker is aware of the problem.

Some clients with persistent depression may benefit from short periods of antidepressive medication, particularly if they are unwilling or unable to talk in depth about the causes of their depression. The main thing is to get the client engaged in constructive activities. Cognitive methods may be helpful: this involves, clients identifying their universally negative self-statements and working on challenging these. They can carry 'cue cards' to remind themselves of the good things about themselves, small or large achievements that they are proud of; turning down a free hit from a friend, for example, or things (other than drugs) which made them feel good. They should identify good times of the day or night to engage in tasks they have identified as constructive.

As part of psychological care, the worker can also reality test and point out the pitfalls of setting goals which are too high, examining the differences between their 'ideal self' and their 'real self'. Many clients will constantly discount any achievements they make, however positive. Sometimes it can be difficult for the worker to think of things the client has achieved: but even turning up for an appointment, managing to have a decent meal, or simply taking only the drugs prescribed for them for one day, going shopping for food, etc., count in this respect. Feelings of being fed up with or sick of the drug scene, if caught at the appropriate moment, can act as a catalyst for change. In the normal run of things, episodes of depression are to be expected, and therapeutic interventions will not always be appropriate or necessary; the client may simply need time to come to terms with their situation. It is the severity of this reaction which the worker needs to be able to gauge. If in doubt it is wise to seek a second opinion from, say, a psychologist or psychiatrist.

Suicide

Clients frequently talk about suicide. It is important that this is discussed in a sensitive manner and to check if the drug user has concrete plans. Clearly, if suicide is discussed with the client it must be made explicit that you are not necessarily condoning the act. If you feel that there is a real threat and that the decision is not being reached in a rational manner, then links with psychiatric support are essential. Unfortunately, this is not always easy, nor is the environment of an in-patient psychiatric ward necessarily the best place for a depressed drug user to be. If you are concerned about the client, particularly if you feel there is a risk of suicide, this should be assessed.

In assessing the risks, ask questions in a straightforward and calm manner. Look for signs, such as giving away personal possessions. Find out if steps have been taken to procure means of committing suicide: has the client been hoarding drugs? Or do they have a significant sum of money with which to procure them? What drugs do they intend to use? If you are concerned and you are not sure, check it out with a colleague. You need to distinguish between suicidal ideas and actual intention, and to gauge the psychological state of the client at the time – rational or irrational – i.e. after a drug binge, under the influence of drugs, tired, confused, deluded, clinically depressed. If the person cannot be persuaded to be admitted to an in-patient unit, compulsory detention may need to be considered. Ultimately, as far as suicide is concerned, we cannot stop people if they are determined. Drug overdose is common among IDU clients and the one question we are often unsure about is, 'Did they mean to do it?': this is a question that affects the worker, the relatives of the deceased and his or her partner and friends. It is a question we are rarely able to answer unless the deceased has made his or her intentions clear. It can leave the bereaved with a sense of shame – the cause of death may not be openly discussed. There can be anger over being rejected as well as guilt – could they have done something to prevent it?: 'If only I'd done more', or 'If only I'd done something different'. The sense of loss and waste can be overwhelming and needs to be acknowledged.

Obsessions and compulsions

Obsessions may take the form of disruptive, repetitive thoughts about illness and death. Compulsions may develop, such as relentlessness searching for symptoms as well as 'displacement activities'. For example, one woman client whose partner was HIV-positive had had two previous negative HIV-antibody tests; her hands used to be raw from the compulsive cleaning of their flat which she would clean until she was exhausted. Symptoms such as these, once identified, may require specialist psychological treatment.

Power

It has to be said that for a group who are marginalised by society, HIV is something that makes people respond (whether positively or negatively). Workers can be galvanised into action. Specialists may want to treat them, researchers to talk to them. Preferential treatment can make people with HIV infection feel special for perhaps the first time in their lives. It is a sad indictment of society's attitudes that only through obtaining a life threatening illness can individuals get this sort of attention. One drug user with AIDS who had got a flat, microwave, washing machine, assistance with bills, and mobility allowance, commented: 'It seems a hell of a price to pay to get a bit of comfort'. It is always advisable to obtain confirmation of a client's diagnosis. One woman was hospitalised for a week before anyone bothered to verify her test result – it turned out to be negative.

References

1. Cushman Jnr., P. & Sherman, C. (1974) Biologic false positive reactions to serologic tests for syphilis in narcotic addiction. *American Journal of Clinical Pathology*, **61**, 346–51.
2. Cushman Jnr., P., Gupta, S. & Grieco, M.H. (1977) Immunological studies in methadone maintained patients. *International Journal of Addictions*, **12**, 241–53.
3. Goodkin, K. (1990) Deterring the progression of HIV infection. *Comprehensive Therapy*, **16**, (8), 17–23.
4. Royce, R.P. & Winkelstein, W. (1990) HIV infection, cigarette smoking and CD4 and T-lymphocyte counts: Preliminary results from the San Francisco Men's Health Study. *AIDS*, **4**, 327–33.
5. Goodkin, K. (1989) A preliminary report of cross-sectional studies of stress, social support and coping style indices in HIV spectrum disorders. *American Association for the Advancement of Science Abstracts*, 51–2.

Chapter 6

Modifying Sexual Behaviour

Introduction

Talking with clients about their sexual behaviour is an important part of the counselling process. In order to be able to provide relevant advice, it is necessary to ask the client some basic questions about their past or present behaviour and relationships. Since sexual behaviour may not be a particular priority for the client – who may be far more concerned with their drug use – this can be easier in theory than in practice.

Sexual counselling issues

Where safer sex is the subject for staff training, either on its own or in combination with other aspects of HIV and AIDS, we are frequently informed that unless we examine our own attitudes and modify our own prejudices, we will not be able to talk openly with our clients about sex. This is a facile argument since it implies that if we attempt to modify our attitudes then it automatically follows that we will be able to counsel competently about sexual behaviour. It does not acknowledge the skills and training required to do sexual counselling. If competent sexual counselling were this easy, then why the need for sex therapists and clinical psychologists to undergo supervised training in this area? This assumption enables us to intellectualise the issues and therefore protect ourselves from our fears and ignorance, 'if I'm broad minded about matters sexual, then I'm a good counsellor about sex'.

Another way of containing our anxieties is by information giving. Although this is an important component of HIV counselling, if it is done in the absence of an accurate and sensitive assessment of the client's situation, then it can lead to feelings of alienation. The counselling process needs to take account of the fact that two individuals (at least) are involved in sexual behaviour. If the client does not enjoy sex, but their partner wants sex, then the client may want to get sex over and done with as quickly as possible. To know the quality and motivation behind the activity is important: each partner may have a different view of this.

There is no point in the client having a stockpile of 'really useful phrases' for use when negotiating safer sex if you are going to get your head kicked in as soon as you mention it to your partner. If you are not likely to see the client again, and they are halfway out of the door, then, 'would you like to take some condoms with you' may be the most practical approach you can take. However, most of us do not work in this barber shop scenario and we frequently see clients again. Our ingenuity to make safer sex meaningful for the client is therefore continuously challenged.

Presumably if we had wanted to become sex therapists that is what we would have become and there are limits to what we should expect of ourselves, given the context of our work. But if we have decided that it is we who have the responsibility to enable clients to reduce their risks of HIV then we must attempt to do this. Appropriate training will therefore be required. Unfortunately, the word 'training', like counselling, contains an infinite amount of variability in terms of content, style, quality, duration and intensity.

Cranfield *et al.*[1] observed in their survey of HIV and drugs training that the issue of safer sex was the one that provoked most embarrassment and the greatest degree of resistance from trainees, especially on courses which opted to use participatory forms of learning. Skills are often the area most neglected.

Training requires a skills-based approach to learning which is situation-specific. The social context of sexual interaction must also be taken into account: there must be a social situation for sexual intercourse to take place; it requires a minimum of two people who may well have very differing views on what they want/do not want to do; what takes place will be affected by the substances injected either before or during the whole process; where and how long they have known the person; the quality of the relationship; the partner's personal knowledge, and power imbalances.

Ideally, the training component should be built into each agency and be on an ongoing basis. If 'in house' trainers are available, i.e. as a unit, or as a local resource, then there is greater possibility for a proactive approach to the content of training rather than one which is reactive – put in place once the problem has emerged.

We hear a great deal about drug users' reluctance to engage in a dialogue with us about their sexual behaviour. Until we as workers are able to develop comfort in talking to each other and to our clients about these sensitive subjects, then our clients will be reluctant to talk to us about sex.[2]

How would it make us feel to be asked by a person who does not provide details of their own personal preferences 'how often do you have sex?' 'what things do you enjoy doing?' 'you may need to stop doing the things you enjoy because they may be dangerous.' How does it feel to be in the position the clients are in when they come to talk to you?

Some drug agencies can be very sexist environments and, frequently, staff have to field comments from clients that they find personally offensive. This is where the educational process can begin – as constructively as possible – in order that clients are not able to use sexism as a defence (or weapon). We should try to ensure that such attitudes are worked with and examined. This is certainly not an easy situation to cope with, however, and, for the counsellor, best not undertaken alone. As an example, how do we introduce the subject of safer sex to clients we have known for years and who misinterpret this as an invitation for physical intimacy? How do we talk to someone of different culture, race and/or sexual preference? These are examples of questions and problems that have become increasingly apparent and that go beyond attitudinal change and consciousness raising.[2]

Answers to certain questions about sexual issues are often not available in textbooks and ignorance about these issues is often difficult for the worker to admit to. It is more difficult to counsel opposite sex clients? It can be, especially if the client who is unused to this subject being discussed in a drug agency setting, misinterprets the counselling as a 'come on' or sets out to exploit the situation. The counsellor needs to be able to defuse this potentially very uncomfortable situation. What do you say if the client asks you, 'Do you use condoms?' This situation is threatening because many of us have not faced up to the need for safer sex in our own lives, or, if we have, we still find it an emotive subject. In other words, it confronts us with our own hypocrisy.

Behaviour changes, once in place, may lapse over time. If the client decides to use safer sex there is no guarantee that this will be applied to all of their current relationships or for all relationships in the future. The possibility is that the behaviour will revert back over time; counselling about safer sex therefore needs to be ongoing. Too often clients respond, 'well, I'm not having sex so it doesn't apply to me', especially just after a diagnosis of being HIV-positive. Invariably, this situation changes as people adjust and become sexually active again so the counselling needs to be appropriate to the current circumstances of the person you see. Planning for the future with an individual who lives for the present is not easy, but should not be abandoned as hopeless.

Promoting safer sexual practices

In basic terms, this means avoidance of sexual activity which involves direct contact of body fluids like blood, semen and vaginal secretions with the lining of the vagina, rectum, penis or non-intact skin.

Although, superficially, the definition may seem fairly straightforward, many different interpretations are possible. For example, when clients at St Mary's were asked in 1990 what they thought the term safer sex meant, 58% mentioned condoms, 25% said 'no casual sex' and 38% mentioned selectivity. This selectivity was primarily in terms of fewer sexual partners. It is therefore useful to elicit what the client thinks safer sex is and their reasoning for this.

The first thing to assess is the individual's sexual behaviour and level of risk. You may not feel comfortable about doing a sexual assessment until you have established a rapport with the client. The main thing is not to avoid doing the assessment completely. It may be useful to elicit some of the following information (not necessarily all at once or in this sequence):

- what is your sexual orientation?
- do you have a regular sexual partner?
- how long have you been in this present relationship?
- does your partner use drugs?
- does your partner know what safer sex is?
- what sexual activities do you engage in?
- have you ever used a condom?
- which sexual activities do you use a condom for, e.g. vaginal, oral or anal?
- how would your partner react to the suggestion of condom use?
- do you have any sexual contacts outside your main relationship?
- where and how do you meet your sexual partners?
- how often do you have sex?
- do you perceive yourselves to be at risk as a result of sexual activity?
- what are your preferred sexual activities?
- (if a woman) are there any irregularities in your menstrual cycle?
- have you ever/do you currently use any form of contraception?
- do you have children?

- how fertile do you perceive yourselves to be?
- (if a woman) are you planning to become pregnant?
- have you ever been to a GP or family planning clinic for advice?
- have you ever had/do you currently have sex for money or drugs?
- (if 'yes' to the above) do you work for yourself?
- where do you meet your customers?
- what activities do you engage in with your customers?
- do you use condoms with your customers?
- does this affect your view of condom use with your sexual partner/s?

If possible, it is useful to delay the information giving until you have the necessary details from the client to put that information into a realistic framework for them. A mediating variable, linked to reduction of risk, is the extent to which individuals expect that preventative behaviour will produce a positive outcome and perceive themselves as capable of enacting preventative practices.[3,4] Adoption of safer sex requires that the person perceives themselves to be at risk from HIV.[4] Since many IDUs do not perceive themselves to be at risk from sexual behaviour, the worker's task is made increasingly difficult.

Although many clients report that their drug use has an adverse effect on their sexual activity, many are still regularly sexually active. Most report a lack of interest as the main sexual problem, although they also report not being particularly bothered by this. Drug use may be the client's first priority, i.e. getting money for drugs, obtaining the drugs, and taking them. Asking clients to adopt safer sex practices is asking them to make major changes in an area of their lives which is not necessarily of major importance to them. It is more likely that changes in drug taking, rather than counselling, will have a significant influence on sexual behaviour and its modification.

There is often a disparity between sexual identity and sexual behaviour; it is important to bear this in mind during an assessment of sexual behaviour.

Condoms

It is not the first time that the condom has had a dual role, both preventing conception and transmission of infection. During the world wars they were issued to soldiers in order to reduce the spread of sexually transmitted diseases. An intact condom will provide an effective barrier for potentially infectious body fluids like semen, vaginal secretions and blood. There is now a wider variety of condoms available with variations in shape, size, colour, thickness, lubrication, taste and scent. Thicker condoms have been produced for extra reliability, both for anal and vaginal intercourse.

Obviously, the condom will only provide protection if it remains intact. According to the UK Family Planning Association, all reliable research shows incorrect usage to be the most significant factor in causing condom failure; used properly, the failure rate is as low as 2%.

So how does one go about choosing? Fortunately, by now, many drug agencies give out condoms free, but the choice is often limited by financial constraints (as is also the case in family planning clinics). If you go into a shop to try to choose, you are often presented with a daunting array of the various types, to say nothing of the expense. Furthermore, what is not clear from many of the packs is exactly the type of condom you are buying. It takes a brave soul to stand and study each pack in detail and even then the necessary information is not always available. This choice also requires the ability to read and to know in advance about things like different types of lubrication.

On the basis of research at St Mary's, those few clients who report using condoms seem to judge the need for condom use with a sexual partner on the basis of how well they knew the person, or, failing that, their appearance. They were slightly more likely to be used with casual rather than with regular partners.

From the 1990 survey, feelings about condoms indicate a general dislike (60% report dislike or intense dislike). Most of the clients expressing dislike were men; those expressing like or neutral feelings were women.

There are various reasons for the negative image of the condom. The most obvious is the disruption it causes in sexual activity. Men also complain of the reduced sensitivity they experience as a result of their use. There may be much awkwardness at the first few attempts at using them and practice and persistence are required. This is incongruent with the popular mythology that sex should be unplanned and spontaneous. There is also the messy task of getting rid of them as soon as possible after ejaculation. Furthermore, suggesting their use can be interpreted either as an admission that you have HIV, or as a lack of trust in your partner. The negative image of condoms thus discourages their use. Although 11% reported that they had never used a condom, they still expressed views on dislike or failure. This is despite a very clear recognition of the value of condoms for protecting against HIV infection (76%). However, generally, the negative image seems to persist.[5]

Our own research picked up accounts of a few men who said they had changed to condom use. They generally told of how they had been forced to adopt safe sex by an assertive, non-drug using partner. One client said that his partner had refused to have sex with him unless he used a condom. These men described their attitudes beforehand as believing that condoms ruined sex, but after a few months they had adapted to the change and now felt neutral about their use; one man even liked using them.[6] The mythology around condoms and bad sex is not necessarily related to experience. Reliable use of the condom as a barrier will also need to be weighed up against the desire to have a child.

In our society, women are frequently made to feel uncomfortable about acknowledging and satisfying their sexual needs. If the man expects the woman to take responsibility for condom use, that woman will have to have them readily available for when they are needed. Many women are still not comfortable about carrying condoms because it implies they are expecting to have sex. This projects what the woman feels to be an unacceptable image of sexual availability. It also suggests that much of the onus for contraception use still lies with the woman. Not only does she have to take responsibility for protecting herself, but for protecting her sexual partner also. In a study of 211 IDUs in New York, condom use was found to be independently associated with greater personal acceptance of condoms. Greater partner receptivity is a factor that is not given sufficient emphasis if the worker focuses solely on the woman's role in contraceptive use.[7]

There have been suggestions that condoms could be marketed to women on feminine hygiene shelves or that the emphasis should be on protection from cervical cancers and provided when attending well woman clinics for check-ups and smear tests. The female condom (worn inside the vagina) is being developed and may soon become commercially available. It is suggested that this will offer an option for the woman. It is unlikely that using it will avoid the need for negotiation with a prospective partner but this remains to be seen. It seems that we are willing to go to extraordinary lengths to ensure that the burden of initiating contraceptive use still remains with the woman. If the woman has to take the lead in suggesting condom use, then she must feel confident about asserting her needs. In order to do this she will both require a healthy level of self esteem and to acknowledge the importance of caring for herself. A chronic problem facing drug users is their low levels of self esteem, even more so among women who use drugs. The emotional, social, economic and political context for the woman needs to be recognised, i.e. how she feels about herself and about caring for herself; her communication skills; her means of financial support; the kind of relationship she is in; the attitudes of her sexual partner, and the stigmatised image that drug users, and particularly women drugs users, have in our society.

The condom also provides a barrier for people working as prostitutes; this can be an advantage as it provides both a physical and psychological barrier between them and their customers, but it makes it more difficult for prostitutes to use condoms in their personal relationships because they are associated with their 'punters' and this cheapens the quality of their personal relationships. As one client put it, her partner would feel she was 'rejecting his sperm'.[6]

Lubricants

For contraceptive purposes, it is recommended that a spermicide be used together with the condom. This extra lubricant should either be put into the vagina or over the outside of the condom when it is on the penis (the contraceptive effectiveness of the condom is 95 to 98% if used with a spermicide, i.e. its efficiency as a method for avoiding pregnancy is enhanced).

Spermicides containing nonoxynol-9 have also been found to have a viricidal action against HIV. It has been used as a lubricant since it can provide added protection should the condom split or come off. Anecdotal evidence from clients suggests that they are unlikely to follow this advice for vaginal sex since it can add to the preparations involved in using a condom. However, some women reported that they liked using it because if they were not sufficiently aroused to be naturally lubricated, the spermicide made sex less uncomfortable for them. Many drug agencies still stock only condoms, without spermicidal lubricants.

For women who suffer from a vaginal inflammation and discharge caused by trichomonas infection, nonoxynol-9 will exacerbate this. When this infection is properly treated and the inflammation clears up, spermicide use should cause no further problems. A very few women report an allergic reaction to nonoxynol-9. Symptoms include a burning sensation, numbness, increased incidence of thrush, and discharge.

Nonoxynol-9 also has an unpleasant taste and one client complained that it ruined her nail varnish! It has been suggested that the tiny ulcerations caused as a result of this adverse response might increase the likelihood of HIV transmission. If there is an allergic reaction then the client could try changing to other types of spermicide or the use of a water-based lubricant, such as KY Jelly which will not have either the spermicidal or viricidal action.

Anal intercourse

An American review of surveys of sexual practices suggests that heterosexual anal intercourse is more common than is generally realised; more than 10% of American women and their male partners engage in the activity with some regularity.[7] Considerably more heterosexuals engage in anal intercourse than do homosexual or bisexual men, not all of whom participate in anal coitus. According to Voeller,[7] anal intercourse carries an HIV risk for women greater than that for vaginal intercourse, just as receptive anal intercourse carries a very high risk for males. Many workers find it difficult to talk about anal sex with their clients. Obviously it is important that they do so, regardless of the client's sexual orientation.

Incidentally, extra lubrication is necessary for anal intercourse in order to facilitate entry of the penis into the rectum. Initially, nonoxynol-9 was recommended as a lubricant because of its viricidal action should the condom split. Condoms tend to have a higher failure rate during anal intercourse. However, it has been reported that nonoxynol-9 causes irritation of the rectal mucosa (lining of the rectum). As a result of the inflammation, there would be an increased blood supply to the area. This would raise the probability of rupture of the blood vessels in the rectum and thus increase the risks of HIV transmission should the condom burst. It is therefore suggested that KY Jelly be used instead. People should be aware that they need to try out different lubricants and spermicides until they find one that suits them and their partner. Oil-based lubricants such as Vaseline and baby oil will weaken the rubber of the condom and can also cause irritation of the rectal mucosa. The use of body fluids such as semen or saliva as lubricants should also obviously be avoided.

Oral sex

The caution about the safety of oral sex is based on the risk of direct contact with possibly infected body fluids such as semen, vaginal secretions and blood in saliva; there is increased risk of exposure if cuts are present on the mouth, lips or genitals.

There have been isolated case reports of HIV transmission via oral sex in the absence of any other apparent risk activity.[8] However, these do not constitute an adequate sample and doubts remain about the reliability of evidence gathered in this way.

HIV antibodies can be found in low concentrations in the saliva of people infected with HIV. There is no evidence that saliva in itself is a viable route of transmission. Indeed, there is also some indication that saliva may inhibit the infectivity of HIV.[9] However, when we asked clients (in 1989/90) about transmission of HIV via saliva, 21% agreed that it could be transmitted via this route.[10] Clearly, there is still some confusion about this.

A similar confusion exists around the potential for HIV to be transmitted during oral sex: 44% agreed with the statement 'oral sex is a high risk activity', for instance. Undoubtedly, we are still uncertain about the relative safety of oral sex. One only has to examine the range of leaflets containing conflicting information about safer sex in order to see how these confusions might arise. Information is often vague and sometimes contradictory. One leaflet, for example, instructs the reader: 'oral sex is probably best avoided until more is known'; another describes oral sex as a 'low risk activity'. A further quote – 'encourage the person to avoid high risk activities such as oral sex'.

Some of the scenarios the client is advised to consider in the various leaflets include the following:

- avoid if there are cuts or sores on the person's mouth/genitals;
- avoid if there are bleeding gums;
- avoid ejaculation into the mouth;
- spit semen out if ejaculation does occur;
- avoid cleaning teeth beforehand (the gums often bleed after cleaning teeth).

Despite the confusion and the lack of feasibility of some of the advice, clients need to weigh up the pros and cons for themselves and their partner(s) and decide whether or not they want to have oral sex.

If a condom is used for oral – penile sex, condoms without spermicidal lubricant are preferable due to normally unpleasant taste of the spermicide – scented or flavoured varieties are available. For oral – vaginal sex, suggestions include the use of dental dams which are thin sheets of latex (about six inches square). The dental dam is placed over the entrance to the vagina in order to prevent direct contact. A small amount of lubricant – e.g. KY Jelly – is put on the side of the dam that is to be in contact with the vagina: this facilitates adhesion and enhances sensitivity. Dental dams have also been suggested for use during oro-anal sex. More creative endeavours have included the use of 'safer sex pants' and clingfilm. The client should be enabled to assess the level of risk for themselves and decide what precautions (if any) they wish to take.

Other sexual practices

Other sexual activities should be assessed in relation to the risks of penetration, tissue damage and body fluid contact involved. There is obviously the potential for developing more creative alternatives to penetrative sex. If the worker his or herself believes this to be the case, then it is probably more likely that the client will be enabled to consider them.

Masturbation

Masturbation and mutual masturbation are considered to be safe activities. Frottage – rubbing the genitals against the intact skin of the partner – is also considered to be safe.

Watersports

This is the term used for urinating onto a partner or into the partner's body. If into a partner's body then penetration may occur. While the urine itself does not constitute a risk, unprotected penetration should be avoided.

Sharing sex toys

Dildos, vibrators or other objects inserted anally or vaginally, will carry the body fluids of the person on whom they were used. If these are shared, there is a potential transmission risk. They should either be kept separate or cleaned properly before each use. One client got around this by putting a condom on her vibrator which she replaced before using it with her partner.

Fisting (inserting hand into anus)

This activity often causes bleeding of the anus or rectal lining. As an isolated activity it is probably relatively low risk provided the skin on the hand of the inserter is intact. However, this activity rarely occurs in isolation and is usually followed by anal intercourse.

Rimming (mouth to anus)

Transmission of HIV via this route is unlikely unless there is bleeding in the mouth or anus. This activity is known to spread gut infections such as *Giardia lamblia* and hepatitis B which may be dangerous to the immunocompromised individual. Use of a barrier such as the dental dam will avoid this risk.

The practice of safer sex contradicts one of our biggest myths about sexual activity – that sex should be spontaneous. Overcoming this belief is a major obstacle to change. The worker needs to establish what the client's expectations of sex and of relationships are.

Barrier, natural, surgical and hormonal contraception

Back-up contraceptive use

Some authorities advise heterosexual women to use a back-up form of contraception if they clearly want to avoid pregnancy (in case the condom should fail). Few women I have seen thus far adhere to this.

According to research carried out at St Mary's Hospital over a five-year period, there has been no significant change in the types of contraceptive used. Overall, contraceptive use remains low.[10] Of the methods available, the pill is the most widely used. Condom use has increased only slightly. In particular, with casual partners, there has been a slight increase in condom use, but not with regular partners. Almost all of the drug users interviewed were in their reproductive years. Of women in the 1985 study, 81% reported menstrual problems, as did 84% of women in the most recent study.[10] Amenorrhoea and irregularity of menses as a result of drug use are the most common complaints. This factor is obviously going to influence the perceived importance of contraceptive use. Many women considered their fertility to be low as a result of their amenorrhoea and most women in the 1990 sample considered pregnancy as moderately or extremely unlikely for them. When asked, over half of women stated that they would like to become pregnant. In the same study, when women who desired to have children were removed from the calculation, 42% of women were using contraceptives consistently (mostly the pill and condom). Contraceptive choice firstly depends on whether or not the client wants to become pregnant. In the USA it was found that the majority of women in drug treatment did not desire more children immediately after giving birth but despite this they also failed to practise effective contraception.[11]

Contraceptive choices are still fairly limited and all carry inherent advantages and disadvantages. Overall, regular use of contraception among IDUs is low. Any advice given must be tailored to the lifestyle of the individual, i.e. what is practical and feasible, and take into account the context in which it will be used – what is the necessary and likely level of co-operation from their partner and the type of relationship the couple are in? If feasible, and if both partners want it, then both of them should be involved in the discussions. The client should be enabled to make a conscious, informed decision. Sometimes the 'choices' are made in less than ideal circumstances: Sue, for example, was due for an operation for termination of pregnancy and was asked just before the operation if she wanted to have a coil fitted. Initially, she said 'yes' and then changed her mind, but in her anxiety before the operation, she forgot to say this. She now has the coil in place and has not bothered to have it removed. It could be argued that this decision was not reached as a result of a fully informed examination of the options. Choice of contraception will also depend on efficiency of the chosen method, i.e. the degree to which pregnancy is avoided. A common way of calculating this is by use of the pregnancy 'Pearl' index. This is calculated as follows.

$$\frac{\text{The number of pregnancies} \times 1200}{\text{Total months of exposure to pregnancy}}$$

You may also see the relative efficiency of a contraceptive expressed as the number of pregnancies per hundred 'women years'; this means the likelihood of pregnancy in 100 women using this method for one year. Some of the contraceptive options available are outlined below.

Natural methods

Abstinence

This is an option that many people insist they will adopt, particularly just after diagnosis of a positive antibody test. If the client is insistent, it can make discussion about safer sex and contraceptive choices very difficult. What tends to happen is that as time goes on the client does become sexually active again. Basically what the worker is attempting to do is to get the client to plan for the future. It is therefore necessary for ongoing discussions to take place. It is also likely that the first incident of renewed sexual intercourse will be closely associated with drug use. Unfortunately, this often means that you see the client after the event. Advice on safer sex then has to be combined with help to overcome their guilt feelings because they have had unsafe sex during this encounter.

Rhythm methods

These methods involve abstaining from sex during the woman's fertile period. They can be complicated to practise because the woman's cycle has to be carefully monitored and this requires a high level of co-operation. Such methods have an effectiveness rate of 80% or more with careful use. I have yet to encounter a client who uses these methods.

Surgical methods

Sterilisation

Early on in the AIDS epidemic, some men were encouraged to have a vasectomy under the mistaken assumption that this measure would eliminate the virus since semen would no longer be produced. Clearly, this is not the case since the virus is present in seminal and pre-ejaculate fluid. Women who have not had children and are not in stable relationships are unlikely to be offered sterilisation as an option because the operation is not readily reversed if they change their minds. These methods are usually 100% effective. A number of HIV-positive women have considered sterilisation. I know of one client who got as far as the operating table and then asked her doctor for reassurance; his rather abrupt retort, that there was never going to be a cure for AIDS, distressed her somewhat so she arose, got up from the operating table, and walked! Many clients feel that the finality of this method is unacceptable.

Hormonal methods

The contraceptive pill

This method has the lowest failure rate. The side effects can include increases in blood pressure and liver problems. It should therefore be borne in mind that not only the lifestyle, but the type of drugs that the woman uses may have an effect in conjunction with the pill, e.g. amphetamines will increase blood pressure; barbiturates make the liver break down the pill more quickly. It should be remembered that if the liver is getting rid of the pill too quickly, this may reduce its efficiency. Antibiotic treatments and heavy diarrhoea also decreases the efficiency of the pill.

There is little information of the effect of the pill on the immune status of the HIV-positive woman. Recent data on the effects of pregnancy on HIV disease progression, however, have been reassuring with respect to hormonal methods. Some studies suggest that the combined pill may increase transmission rates.[12,13] The mechanism proposed for this is that the pill increases susceptibility to infection either by changing the composition of the surface cells of the vagina and cervix or through cell mediated immunity. This is not yet proven and further investigation is required.[14,15,16]

The pill needs to be taken regularly in order to be an effective contraceptive. The combined pill has an effectiveness rate of 100%; the mini-pill (or progesterone-only pill) has an effectiveness rate of 98 to 99%. Some forms of the mini-pill even require that they be taken within a four-hour limit. There is the added advantage of less bleeding with the mini-pill, although this may occur irregularly.

Many IDUs do not have a well-regulated, organised lifestyle. Of those women who have chosen to use the pill, many were taking it inconsistently but were still relying on this as their main form of contraception (possibly as a result of their low perceived fertility). Taking the pill can also cause problems for the person who wants to avoid pregnancy, but also practice safer sex. Many women feel that it is easier for them not to use any form of contraception so that they can avoid complicated explanations with their partners as to why they feel the need to use the pill as well as a condom. This problem also arose in the case of a recently diagnosed HIV-positive man who wanted to use condoms. He was not yet ready to tell his partner (who was on the pill) that he was HIV-positive as he was afraid that she would leave him as a result. His compromise was to tell her that he had talked to a drug worker about HIV; he did not want to have the test done just yet, but, to be on the safe side, would she mind if they used condoms as well. Fortunately, she agreed to this.

The morning-after pill can be an effective contraceptive for up to three days after intercourse has taken place. It is therefore useful in cases where no contraception has been used and the woman wants to avoid pregnancy; however, it has no benefit as far as HIV transmission in concerned.

Injectable method

This method keeps a low but effective level of artificial hormone in the body. The effect of drug interactions with this method are also relevant. The hormonal injection method has the advantage that it provides contraceptive protection for three to six months which is useful since it means that the woman can forget about contraception for the effective duration of the injection or implant – it is almost 100% effective. Unfortunately, this also means that a lot of women forget when their next injection is due and it can take an extended period of time before they can get their next injection organised. This situation can be greatly improved if a family planning doctor or GP is available to do these injections when the client attends a drug agency. Obviously, this type of service has resource implications and is more likely to be available to drug agencies within an NHS setting.

The disadvantage of this method is that it interferes with the menstrual cycle – a significant number of women cease menstruation or have irregular periods as a result (although reduced bleeding may be beneficial with respect to HIV risk). This disadvantage may be minimised among women who suffer from extended periods of amenorrhoea. It becomes more significant when the woman either comes off drugs or stabilises on methadone. To women at such times, the reappearance of their periods is sometimes seen as a strong positive indication that their body is returning back to 'normal'. Other women feel that their periods are necessary for 'cleaning out' every month (although this is not in fact the case). Weight gain and depression have also been associated with this method. If a women has the injection she cannot change her mind for the three-month period and return of fertility may be delayed. However, despite these disadvantages many clients find this a convenient method to use and appreciate the low level of participation it requires from them.

Barrier methods

Diaphragm or cap

The vaginal cap consists of a thin rubber dome which fits inside the vagina behind the pelvic bone and covers the cervix. Smaller forms of 'barrier' caps are also available which fit directly over the cervix. This method may serve to protect the cervix which is well supplied with blood vessels. It is probably protective against cervical cancer, but is not sufficient for protection against HIV since the vaginal walls are still exposed. It has the advantage that it is used in combination with spermicide, especially if the spermicide contains the viricidal agent nonoxynol-9 (the problems with adverse reactions to this have already been discussed). It is 97 to 98% effective as a contraceptive.

However, this method requires a lot of motivation and advance organisation. Should the woman decide that she wants to have intercourse she needs to have the cap and spermicide readily available in order to fit it beforehand. More spermicide needs to be inserted each time intercourse takes place. This may prove daunting if used in conjunction with a condom as well. The other factor that needs to be considered is that women who are experiencing excessive weight loss of more than 2–3 lbs due to HIV-related causes will need to have their cap refitted as the size may need to be altered.

The spermicidal sponge is not widely used as yet by the women we have seen – it has low reliability and should not be relied on as an effective contraceptive.

The coil or inter-uterine device (IUD)

The coil or IUD has the advantage that it can be forgotten about once it is in place. It is 97 to 98% effective. However, HIV-positive women are advised against its use because of the associated infection risk, e.g. pelvic inflammatory disease and actinomycosis infection.[17] There is a risk of fungal infection with long-term use. It is advisable to avoid infections of this nature because they may act as co-factors to HIV disease progression. There does not yet appear to be any systematic evaluation of this risk, which is unfortunate, since the coil is a potentially useful method, given the ease of its use. It is not usually advised for women who have not had children. The disadvantage of heavy and painful periods is largely avoided if the woman has amenorrhoea but not otherwise, and heavy bleeding will be a disadvantage where HIV risk is concerned. If periods return they can be painful.

A major disadvantage of this method is that many IDU women forget to have their coil checked until complications arise. Missed appointments can mean long delays before the client and the doctor are in the same place at the same time. For one of my clients it took a full year of failed attempts before we achieved our goal and she was examined (her coil had been fitted three years previously). Another client suffered from severe stomach cramps and vaginal discharge but still missed her appointments. Eventually she pulled the infected coil out herself and then went for a check-up.

If the woman is in the later stages of AIDS then increased menstrual loss may exacerbate anaemia. It has also been suggested that the string from the coil may lacerate a penis or condom during sex, thus creating a transmission risk.[18] This risk has not been systematically evaluated and remains a 'theoretical possibility'.

Sexual transmission risks

Sexual transmission through intercourse with an infected man is most likely to occur through infected lymphocytes in the ejaculate, free virus in the seminal fluid, or through immune complexes consisting of HIV particles, ineffective antibodies, and complement. There is now evidence that as the HIV-positive person's immune system declines, they become more infectious. HIV in seminal fluid appears to increase with advancing disease, and in men with genital tract infection (GTI).[19] Spermatazoa may not harbour HIV and a man may not consistently shed virus into his semen. Anderson *et al.* found HIV in the semen of men with early infections and in men with no GTI. De Vincenzi[20] suggests that a man with AIDS is three times more likely to infect his female partner than a man who is HIV-positive but with no symptoms.

T-cell depletion has been shown to be a major determinant in infectivity.[21] The immune system may also play a role in protecting the partner from HIV infection. If the partner's immune system is already poor due to ill health and poor nutrition, then they may be more susceptible. This emphasises the need for good overall health for drug users.

It might be expected that long duration of relationship and a high frequency of sexual intercourse would increase the risks of transmission, but several studies have failed to demonstrate this.[22,23,24] Two studies have described cases where transmission occurred from male to female following one or two acts of sexual intercourse.[22,24]

Risk of acquiring HIV from a single heterosexual contact with an infected person is not fully known. However, the risk of transmission during a single sexual exposure has been estimated from studies of the heterosexual partners of HIV-infected people to be between 0.001 and 0.01 per sexual contact.[25]

Advising HIV-discordant couples

This term is applied to couples where one partner in HIV-antibody-positive and the other is negative. Where HIV-discordant couples do not practise safer sex, delayed seroconversion in the negative partner can facilitate their belief that it will not happen to them, particularly in the absence of illness or physical evidence in the HIV-positive partner. 'Well, if that's the case, why am I still negative?' 'I believe that I can't catch it.' Inventing theories, 'maybe I've got a strain that isn't infectious', 'I don't think the virus is going to go any further'.

The other reaction we have observed is that not practising safer sex is a way of declaring your regard for your positive partner. Tina and Pat were a couple who knew each other years ago and took up their relationship again. Tina was HIV-positive. They were not having safer sex although her partner was fully aware of her HIV status. 'He says he doesn't mind.' Any possible consequences were far removed from the present. Neither of them felt the need to prevent this vague and non-evident HIV. This reaction is more evident when the HIV-positive partner is asymptomatic, presumably because AIDS is still a remote possibility in the future and the denial process can operate more effectively.

Even when a couple adopt safer sex initially, as the relationship develops they can forget about their past and issues of trust and intimacy take precedence over the need for safer sex. Whatever the couple's response to HIV, both partners face the consequences either directly or indirectly. Even when safer sex is practised by the couple, it can present its own problems. One HIV-positive man commented, 'I don't know why we both bother (to have sex); I get up immediately, tie a knot in the condom, go to the bathroom and make sure it's flushed down the toilet. It's all so clinical, I don't think my wife enjoys sex anymore, and it reminds me about the virus. The other reaction observed is where the negative partner becomes fearful of having sex. This can occur even when couples are practising safer sex: Heather, for example, expressed profound relief that her HIV-positive partner did not want sex. 'I try to hide it, but I'm sure he knows how frightened I am; we take all the precautions that we can, but I just can't help being afraid.'

Heather also used to encourage her partner not to reduce his methadone dosage in the hope that the drug would curtail his desire for sex. A further implication of this is that if the sexual relationship breaks down, people may not try to sort this out because of the relief they feel that they no longer have to have sex. In an example of this, Claire was quite content to stay with her partner although he had told her that he wanted the relationship to finish. She could cope better with a platonic relationship and she had no other accommodation to go to. At the same time the situation was damaging to her self esteem since he had rejected her.

Another non-drug using woman could cope only by going away on her own to stay with friends and leaving her positive partner to look after the children. This left him feeling very resentful but she felt she needed the space.

Waiting for illnesses or watching out for them can put a terrible strain on the relationship. The negative partner also has to cope with the fear and sometimes anger about their partner's status. There may be children involved and fear about how the family will cope if and when the infected partner dies.

Prostitution

Much has been written about prostitutes and the potential they have to transmit HIV, particularly in the case of drug-using prostitutes. It has been suggested that drug-using prostitutes will be less likely to use condoms with their customers. It is also suggested that the drug-using prostitutes will be more vulnerable to customer demands, that the need for money for drugs will override the desire for safer sex if they are offered more money for not using a condom. In some areas of the UK it has been observed that competition for clients may lead drug-using prostitutes to take greater risks for customers, and may interfere with prudent patterns of work, e.g. not going off in a car alone with two or three men.[26] However, this contrasts with reports of regular condom use among drug-using prostitutes in other studies.[27,28]

In the St Mary's study all the women working as prostitutes carried condoms; most of whom expressed anxiety about carrying them due to police harassment. The evidence is patchy and frequently contradictory. The problem for many of the studies is access to adequate numbers of drug-using women who work as prostitutes; data on male prostitutes is even more scant. There is in fact virtually no scientifically adequate data on male prostitutes.

There appears to be a group of women and men drug users who may intermittently engage in prostitution as a source of funding for drugs. As a result of the intermittent nature of this activity, they may be more likely to take risks (not only in terms of HIV transmission) and less likely to care for their sexual health – they may not perceive themselves to be professional prostitutes. The 'occasional freelancer' is still likely to have a drug user as a sexual partner so the risk for this group are very difficult to assess.

Many drug-using prostitutes will also have sexual partners who are drug users themselves. There is therefore a dual risk of infection via shared injecting equipment and sexual transmission. They are less likely to use condoms with their regular sexual partners. Prostitution may be the sole financial support for their own and their partner's habit.

According to Padian,[29] research among women working as prostitutes has indicated a distinct trend towards not using condoms with their regular sexual partners, or indeed some long-term regular clients, due to their qualitatively different relationships. A different approach to safer sex will be required in order that condoms are not used to distinguish customers from lovers. Love and trust do not foster condom use. There is some indication that drug use may be a more important factor in HIV transmission that a drug-using partner or than multiple partners.

In three separate surveys among intravenous drug abusers, prostitution was not an independent risk factor for HIV.[30,31,32] Needle sharing practices in different locations will influence the level of HIV in the community of those engaged in prostitution.

In the 1990 study conducted at St Mary's,[5] prostitution accounted for only 6% of the funding for drugs. Shoplifting and employment (mostly casual labour) constituted the two major sources of income for drugs (30% and 24% respectively). In a 1985 study,[33] 15 clients (20%) reported at some time having sex for drugs or money (a broad definition of prostitution). In the 1990 sample, 31% of clients reported that they had at some time engaged in prostitution as a source of funding for their drugs. However, only 12% reported current work. Over half of those who worked professionally had been offered more money by their customers for not using condoms. Recent research suggests that power may be an important factor in motivating men to seek sex with prostitutes, because the interaction allows the man to assume that he can 'do anything'.[34,35]

There is anecdotal evidence that women who are recruited into prostitution who have a drug habit, or women who acquire a drug habit after becoming prostitutes, may have a somewhat shorter career than those who do not use drugs. In the United States there are reports of women becoming the semi-permanent residents of 'crack houses'. Crack use often results in increased violence and sexual risk-taking on the women's part.

The nature of the work may expose the prostitute to pressure to use drugs. One IDU working for an escort agency was offered cocaine at most of the 'parties' she went to. Her customers often actively encouraged drug use to enhance the sexual experience.

Sophie, who worked for an escort agency, took Valium in order to cope with her work. She took it just before she went out to work. Her income was declining as she got older and she worried because she had not managed to save her earnings. As to finding a partner – 'most decent blokes would mind about my past, and if they said it didn't matter, I wouldn't respect them anyway'. The prostitute often has limited economic options if she wants to stop working. They are also at a far greater risk of arrest because of having both an illegal drug habit and engaging in prostitution as a source of income.

Sexual abuse and assault

HIV has been reportedly transmitted by heterosexual rape.[36] Due to the physical trauma involved, risk of transmission may be greater under these circumstances. HIV-antibody testing should be offered to a person who has been raped at intervals of three and six months after the assault. The possible role of early AZT treatment to prevent sero-conversion in victims of rape has yet to be clarified. Psychological support should also be available during this period and as long after-wards as the individual requires it.[18]

Many women and some men in the 1990 St Mary's study report having been physically or sexually abused.[1] Of those interviewed, 41% reported that they had at some time been sexually assaulted and over half of these were assaults on women in the last five years. This suggests that women drug users may be more vulnerable to sexual assault in their adult lives, possibly as a result of the lifestyle associated with their drug use. Jan reported that she had been gang raped after leaving her dealer's flat in the early hours of the morning, and sub-sequently wandered through a rough housing estate alone. One im-plication of this is that such incidents are extremely unlikely to be reported to the police.

Advising clients to ask their partners to use condoms can risk further abuse. The decision to use condoms needs to be based on the women's perception of the cost or benefit to that particular relationship and the relationship's role in the woman's economic, social and physical sur-vival. As an example, Josephine's mobility problems were not the result of AIDS. When she was working as a prostitute she attempted to keep some money back from her pimp – he broke both her legs.

Childhood abuse is commonly reported by clients. When she was a teenager, Sue's father would wait for her to come home at night and try to catch her climbing back in through the window. When he caught her he closed the window on her arm and broke it in two places. IDUs also report childhood sexual abuse that occurred when they were staying in children's homes.

One implication of this is that if a worker is going to discuss sexual behaviour with their clients, they will need to be competent to cope with the situation should such sensitive and emotive information be disclosed. This is not to suggest that the worker should be able to do in-depth counselling for those suffering from sexual trauma. What it does mean is that they should have clear lines of referral to therapists who specialise in this work if they feel this is required. Knowing our limitations is very important. A further implication of the effect of sexual abuse on the individual is the devastating effect it can have on the person's self-esteem. If IDU women are left to take the lead in contraception or condom use, then they will need to feel confident about themselves and the need to care for their own bodies. A history of sexual abuse is unlikely to facilitate this attitude.

References

1. Cranfield, S. & Dixon, A. (1990) Drugs training, HIV and AIDS in the 1990's: a guide for training professionals. London: Health Education Authority.
2. Cranfield, S. (1990) Safer sex education with drug users. In *Harm Reduction: Drugs and HIV/AIDS*. (Ed. P.M. Fleming), Wessex Regional Health Authority.
3. Christiansen, B.A. & Goldman, M.S. (1983) Alcohol related expectancies versus demongraphic/background variables in the prediction of adolescent drinking. *Journal of Consulting and Clinical Psychology*, **51**, 245–57.
4. Marlatt, G.A. & Ronsenow, D. (1980) Cognitive processes in alcohol use: expectancy and the balanced placebo design. In *Advances in Substance Abuse: Behavioural and Biological Research* (Ed. N. Mello), JAI Press, New York, 115–36.
5. Mulleady, G. & Cupitt, C. (1991) Sexual issues for women drug users. National Conference on Women and Substance Misuse, London, March 1991.
6. Cupitt, C., Mulleady, G., Phillips, K. & White, D. (1991) Condom use among injecting drug users. Unpublished.
7. Uoeller, B. (1991) AIDS and heterosexual anal intercourse. *Archives of Sexual Behaviour*, **20**, No. 3, 233–76.
8. Perry, S., Jacobsberg, L. & Fogel, K. (1989) Orogenital transmission of human immunodeficiency virus (HIV). *Annals of Internal Medicine* III (II), 951–2.
9. Fox, P.C., Witt, D.J., Yen, C.K., *et al.* (1988) Saliva inhibits HIV I infectivity. *Journal of the American Medical Association*, **116**, 635–7.
10. Mulleady, G., White, D., Phillips, K. & Cupitt, C. (1990) Reducing sexual transmission of HIV for injecting drug users: the challenge for counselling. *Counselling Psychology Quarterly*, **3**, (4), 325–41.
11. Eldred, C.A. & Washington, M.N. (1975) Female heroin addicts in a city treatment programme: the forgotton minority. *Psychiatry*, **38**, 75–85.
12. Johnson, A.M., Petherick, A., Davidson, S.J., *et al.* (1989) Transmission of HIV to heterosexual partners of infected men and women. *AIDS*, **3**, 367–72.
13. Mann, J.M., Nzilambi, N., Piot, P., *et al.* (1988) HIV infection and associated risk factors in female prostitutes in Kinshasa, Zaire, *AIDS*, **2**, 249–54.
14. Jones, L. & Catalan, J. (1989) Women and HIV disease. *British Journal of Hospital Medicine*, **41**, 526–38.

15. Plummer, F.A., Simmonsen, J.N., Ngugi, E.N., Cameron, D.W., Piot, P. & Ndinya-Achola, J.O. (1987) Incidence of human immunodeficiency virus infection and related disease in a cohort of Nairobi prostitutes. III International Conference on AIDS, Washington, June 1987, (Abstract, M8.4).
16. Plummer, F., Cameron, W., Simonsen, N., *et al.* (1988) Co-factors in male-female transmission of HIV. IV International Conference on AIDs. Stockholm June 1988, (Abstract 4554).
17. Safrin, S., Dattel, B.J., Haver, L.B., *et al.* (1989) Prevalence and risk factors for HIV-1 infection in patients with acute pelvic inflammatory disease (PID). V International Conference on AIDS, Montreal, June 1989 (Abstract MBP54).
18. Bradbeer, C. (1990) Human immunodeficiency virus and its relationship to women. International Journal of STD and *AIDS*, **1**, 233–8.
19. White, K. (1990) Artificial insemination and HIV infection: research shows sperm may not harbour the virus. *AIDS Patient Care*, Dec, 25–26.
20. Brown, P. (1990) Sex during periods raises risk of HIV spread. *New Scientist*, 5 May, p. 24.
21. Rowen, D. & Carne, C.A. (1990) Heterosexual transmission of human immunodeficiency virus. *International Journal of STD and AIDS*, **1**, 239–44.
22. Johnson, A.M., Petherick, A., Davidson, S., *et al.* (1989) Transmission of HIV to heterosexual partners of infected men and women. *AIDS*, **3**, 367–72.
23. European Study Group (1989) Risk factors for male to female transmission of HIV. *British Medical Journal*, **298**, 411–5.
24. Peterman, T.A., Stoneburner, R.L., Allen, J.R., *et al.* (1988) Risk of HIV transmission from heterosexual adults with transfusion associated infections. *Journal of the American Medical Association*, **259**, 55–8.
25. Cameron, D.W., Simonsen, J.N., D'Costa, L.J., *et al.* (1989) Female to male transmission of human immunodeficiency virus type 1: risk factors for seroconversion in men. *Lancet*, Aug, 403–7.
26. Rosenberg, M.J. & Weiner, J.M. (1988) Prostitutes and AIDS: a health department priority? *American Journal of Public Health*, **78**, 418–23.
27. Perkins, R. (1985) Aids and prostitution. *British Medical Journal*, **143**, 426.
28. Carmen, A. & Moody, H. (1985) *Working women: the subterranean world of street prostitution*. New York: Harper and Row.
29. Padian, N.S. (1988) Prostitute women and AIDS: epidemiology. *AIDS*, **2**, 412–13.
30. Tirelli, V., Vaccheri, E., Sorio, R., Carbone, A. & Monfardini, S. (1986) HTLV-III antibodies in drug addicted prostitutes used by U.S. soldiers in Italy. *Journal of the American Medical Association*, **257**, 1047.
31. Dan, M., Rock, M. & Bar-Shani, S. (1987) HIV antibodies in drug addicted prostitutes. *Journal of the American Medical Association*, **257**, 1047.
32. Van den Hoek, J.A.R. Coutinho, R.A., Van Haastrecht H.J.A. Van Zadelhoff, A.W. & Goudsmit, J. (1988) Prevalence and risk factors of HIV infection among drug users and drug using prostitutes in Amsterdam. *AIDS* **2**, 55–60.

33. Mulleady, G. & Sherr, L. (1989) Lifestyle factors for drug users in relation to risks for HIV. *AIDS Care*, **1** (1), 45–50.
34. Delacoste, F. & Alexander, P. (1987) *Sex work*: writings by women in the sex industry. Pittsburgh: The Cleis Press.
35. Schedlin, M.G. (1987) If you wanna kiss, go home to your wife: sexual meanings for the prostitute and implications for AIDS prevention activities. Presented at the American Anthropological Association, November.
36. Murphy, S., Kitchen, V., Harris, J.R.W. & Forster, S.M. (1989) Rape and subsequent seroconversion to HIV. *British Medical Journal*, **299**, 718–19.

Chapter 7

Women and HIV

Introduction

By the end of the 1980s there were an estimated 100 000 infected women in Northern America, and 60 000 in Europe with HIV. The late 1980s saw seroprevalence rise rapidly in Thailand and in female prostitutes in several cities in India. An estimated 225 000 women in Africa, and 10 000 women in the USA had developed AIDS by the end of the 1980s.[1] In North America AIDS is already the leading cause of death in women between 20 and 40 years of age.

Predictions of women and children at risk

It is predicted that by the end of 1992, in the African continent, there will be cumulative totals of 4 million women and 1 million children infected by HIV and 600 000 women with AIDS, of whom about one quarter will have developed disease in the year 1992.[2]

Research on the sexual behaviour of women IDUs has concentrated on fertility patterns rather than on their sexuality, i.e. on management of the pregnant drug user, rather than on the care of the drug-using woman. Behavioural research on the relationship between sex and drug use has concentrated on the male subculture, hence the paucity of data on the relationship between female drug use and decision making. Studies of female drug users are rare.[3]

For reasons that are not fully understood, women in the USA and other Western nations are more likely to contract HIV from men rather than to transmit the virus to them through sexual contact.[4,5]

Des Jarlais *et al.*[6] indicated that 80% of male IDUs were in primary relationships with women who did not use drugs. Women are more likely than male IDUs to be directly and indirectly associated with drug use. There is even less knowledge about the non-drug using sexual partners of IDU men.

Women with HIV have been found to have a higher incidence of abnormal cervical cells.[7,8] It has not yet been shown if this leads to symptomatic cervical cancer in HIV-positive women, although there is some evidence that pre-malignant lesions worsen and respond poorly to treatment.[9] It is important for all women, but HIV-positive women especially, to have regular smear tests. Lack of medical care, lack of concern for their own health, and poor attendance, can lead to more serious consequences for the drug-using woman. For example, Cathy found she had seriously abnormal cervical cells only when her pregnancy was discovered. She decided she wanted to risk having the baby because of the possibility of hysterectomy should the results of her cone biopsy show malignancy. She was advised against this decision and therefore had her pregnancy terminated. The results of her biopsy indicated that she did not require the hysterectomy, but the termination was an outcome that might have been avoided had she received regular cervical screening.

Certain HIV-associated illnesses and AIDS may have different manifestations in women. Kaposis's sarcoma is very rare in women or in drug users as a whole although it is more common in African women and those infected by bisexual men.[10] The vaginal incidence of candida (thrush) may be more common than oral and oesophageal candida in HIV-positive women and women with AIDS. There is anecdotal evidence that women given AZT may be less tolerant of it than men. Women have been under-represented in drug trials, and clearly this imbalance needs to be redressed. Other than the differences already mentioned, the disease profile in women seems to be little different from that of men apart from the differences in tumours found in women. More relevant is access to health care, and early diagnosis. HIV- and AIDS-related illnesses in women may be misdiagnosed by health care staff because it may not occur to them to investigate HIV as a possible cause.

Promoting equality in health care

Much attention has been drawn to the need for women to have empowerment but how is this achieved? No one would argue that this needs to happen or deny that it is an ongoing process – chipping away at the inequalities that exist for women in society, but, for many women, empowerment is just a word. Being poor is real. Having children to look after is real. Being afraid of being alone is real.[11]

Oppression occurs on sexual, cultural, political and socio-economic levels. It could be argued that empowerment begins with economic independence. Women who are financially dependent on men or who exchange sex for money or drugs may face the dilemma of choosing between economic survival and unsafe sex.[12,13]

Powerlessness is evident in many of the women's relationships with their male partners even when they are earning the money for both of their drug habits. Worth maintains that women have internalised their powerlessness as a reflection of their own self worth which often leaves them with a feeling of despair, defeatism and fatalism.[12] This fatalism may be seen in the woman's reaction to a positive HIV result or in their response to being battered, e.g. Val would telephone her worker when she had been battered by her partner. She was unable to leave her partner, although other options were open to her. She would regularly turn up to the clinic with teeth missing and black eyes, which gave rise to considerable frustrations for the worker. If a woman feels fatalistic about life, then the impact of the consequences of HIV infection will be lessened. When the more pervasive problems are recognised by both worker and client, then the reasons for the so-called fatalistic or passive attitude that women drug users can have towards HIV become clearer.

Part of the need is to enable men to recognise how much they rely on the woman to care for them and to take responsibility for contraception. They need to be aware of their reactions to women who 'take the lead sexually', for some men this may be a relief, for others it may carry negative connotations in their subsequent attitudes to the woman.

Women IDUs require possibilities to enhance self worth other than through motherhood which is the route many of them take. Frequently the woman IDU is left with sole responsibility of caring for the child, the father's role being confined to his biological contribution. However, until more significant changes are brought about, advantage should be taken of the opportunity to provide a wider range of services in the antenatal setting. Women IDUs are most likely to attend for health care when pregnant. Investment must be made in the maternity services to enable them to play their role in the prevention of HIV transmission, through the dissemination of information, family planning advice, counselling and medical care for HIV-positive women and for women with AIDS. Ante-natal clinics are possible points for the integration of HIV prevention with primary health care.

Lesbian issues

Lesbians are a rarely recognised group in genitourinary medicine[14] and the same could be said for their involvement in HIV and AIDS. There are, however, a number of areas in which they may be affected:

(1) Concern over the safety of oral sex, transmission via vaginal fluids and menstrual blood and confusion about this. Evidence for transmission by oro-genital contact has only been from isolated case studies up to 1989.[15,16] All but one of these involved apparent female to female transmission following a lesbian relationship with an HIV-infected partner. By no means do they constitute a sound or adequate sample, but they do throw some doubt on the absolute safety of oro-genital contact and certainly do not dismiss the risk for lesbians.
(2) Those affected by their drug use.
(3) There is a reported increase in (heterosexual) prostitution among lesbians addicted to crack (in order to finance their habit). Apart from a source of income for drugs, prostitution may be the sole income anyway.
(4) Many lesbians will have had sex with men at some time in their lives. There are anecdotal reports of lesbians becoming infected via this route.
(5) Lesbians may be at risk of HIV infection through artificial insemination. Although donors to semen donor banks are tested for HIV before the semen can be used, unofficial donation may put the woman at risk.[10]
(6) Their caring role is frequently ignored. They are as affected as anyone else by caring for and seeing their friends and relatives die.
(7) They are familiar with discrimination as a result of their sexual preference and therefore can identify with the discrimination gay men and IDUs have received as a result of HIV and AIDS. This discrimination has undoubtedly increased as a result of AIDS hysteria. Their political awareness and experience should be acknowledged.
(8) Little research on those who identify themselves as lesbian or gay has taken place outside the urban communities in which there are

concentrations of potential respondents. Understanding, therefore, is restricted to a few contacts despite evidence that even within countries, sexual lives and networks differ from community to community.[17]

(9) One study found that in lesbians attending an STD clinic, abnormal smear tests were not uncommon.[14] There is a need for lesbians to have regular smear tests, especially if they have had earlier heterosexual intercourse.

References

1. Fleming, A.F. (1990) Implications of AIDS for women and children. *Current AIDS Literature*, **3** (7), 217–18.
2. Chin, J. (1990) Current and future dimensions of the HIV/AIDS pandemic in women and children. *Lancet*, **336**, 221–4.
3. Rosenbaum, M. (1979) Becoming addicted: the woman addict. *Contemporary Drug Problems*, **8**, 141–6.
4. Morbidity and Mortality Weekly Report (1989) Update: Heterosexual transmission of Acquired Immunodeficiency Syndrome and Human Immunodeficiency Virus infection – United States. MMWR, **38**, 423–34.
5. Wiley, J.A. & Herschkorn, S.J. (1989) Heterogeneity in the probability of HIV transmission per sexual contact: the case of male to female transmission in penile–vaginal intercourse. *Statistics in Medicine*, **8**, 93–102.
6. Des Jarlais, D.C., Chamberland, M.E., Yancovitz, S.R., Weinberg, P. & Friedman, S.R. (1985) Heterosexual partners: a large risk group for AIDS. *Lancet*, **2**, 1346–7.
7. Bradbeer, C. (1987) Is infection with HIV a risk factor for cervical intraepithelial neoplasia? *Lancet*, **(ii)**, 1277–8.
8. Byrne, M.A., Taylor-Robinson, D., Munday, P.E. & Harris, J.R. (1989) The common occurance of human papillomavirus infection and intraepithelial neoplasia in women infected by HIV. *AIDS*, **3**, 379–82.
9. Bradbeer, C.S. & Heyderman, E. (1989) The risk of progression of crucial dysplasia in women with HIV. V International Conference on AIDS, Montreal (Abstract MBP 58).
10. Bradbeer, C. (1990) Human immunodeficiency virus and its relationship to women. *International Journal of STDs and AIDS*, **1**, 233–8.
11. Wilson, J. (1988) The role of counselling women and AIDS conference: needs, issues, awareness. Edinburgh, May 1988.
12. Worth, D. (1989) Sexual decision making and AIDS: why condom promotion among vulnerable women is likely to fail. *Studies in Family Planning*, **20**, (6, 1), 297–307.
13. Williams, A. (1985) When the client is pregnant: information for counsellors. *Journal of Substance Abuse Treatment*, **2**, 27–34.
14. Edwards, A. & Thin R.N. (1990) Sexually transmitted diseases in lesbians. *International Journal on STD and AIDS*, **1**, 187–81.

15. Monzon, O.T. & Capellan, J.M.B. (1987) Female to female transmission of HIV. 6 *Lancet* (**ii**), 40.
16. Marmor, M., Weiss, L.R., Lyden, M., Weiss, S.H. & Saxinger, W.C. (1986) Possible female to female transmission of human immunodeficiency virus. *Annals of Internal Medicine*, **105**, 969.
17. White, E. (1980) *States of desire: travels in gay America*. New York: E.P. Dutton.

Chapter 8

Pregnancy, Drug Use and HIV

Introduction

The World Health Organization predicts that by 1992 over one million children worldwide will be infected with HIV.[1] According to Mok, AIDS could be a major cause of death among children by the end of the century.[2]

In North America AIDS is already the leading cause of death in children below the age of four years.[3] Surveys of pregnant women in selected settings have found HIV infection varies from nearly 1% in Paris to 31% in New York City. An estimated 300 000 children in Africa and 12 000 children in the USA had developed AIDS by the end of the 1980s. In Central Africa alone, there will be 5 million orphans by AD 2000 and large numbers are predicted also in the Caribbean and in New York City.[4]

Drug use and fertility

As discussed earlier, most women who use heroin regularly will suffer from amenorrhoea or irregularity of menses. As a result of loss of menstruation, many women believe their fertility to be low. The perceived importance of contraception is thus reduced and the likelihood of so called 'unplanned' pregnancy is increased. This will also adversely affect a pregnant woman's accuracy in estimating the date of conception. Not only will amenorrhoea influence the perceived need for contraceptive use, but also the perceived likelihood of becoming pregnant. Most of the women interviewed in the 1990 study at St Mary's considered pregnancy to be moderately or extremely unlikely.[5]

Opiate and opioid drugs depress the functioning of the hypothalamic system in the brain; this causes a depression in the production of follicle stimulating hormone (FSH) and luteinising hormone (LH), crucial to the control of the reproductive cycle. This can result in lowered fertility.[6,7] Although heroin use can suppress fertility, in some cases, higher birth rates have been found for drug-using women than for non-drug-using women.[8] Although menstruation ceases, ovulation may continue.

In response to regular methadone use in women who have previously used heroin menstruation can recommence. Women can suffer from painful and irregular periods at this time. This probably also coincides with an increase in fertility. Once a woman dependent on opiates begins using methadone, this factor needs to be taken into consideration. Pregnancy may seem a very remote possibility to her, particularly if she has never used contraception before and managed to avoid pregnancy.

Prescribed and non-prescribed drug use during pregnancy

As well as stabilising drug use, if the client is trying to become pregnant it is useful to discuss their nutrition with respect to improving overall health and the chances of conception. Access to a dietitian can be useful when the client becomes pregnant because often IDUs neglect their diet and are frequently under-weight. They may lack basic knowledge about adequate nutrition. If the dietitian has an understanding of the client's lifestyle, this is especially useful because they can then give realistic advice about what to do: cheap and easy-to-prepare foods and ready-made meals, for example. We have found that where nutrition is otherwise inadequate, nutritional or 'liquid food' drinks can be a popular last ditch option.

Despite their being stable on methadone, we have seen a number of HIV-positive couples who want a child and have difficulty conceiving. They have required further counselling and treatment regarding management of their infertility problems and for some practitioners this raises an ethical dilemma, given the risks of HIV transmission to the child. In some cases this had led to HIV-positive couples being turned down for fertility treatment.

The effect of drugs on the fetus is one of the few areas where women drug users have been studied. Obviously, the baby is exposed to the drugs that the pregnant woman takes. The fetal tissues metabolise drugs poorly; what is excreted into the amniotic fluid is re-ingested so that the concentration in fetal tissues can be higher than in maternal tissues. The developing fetus has to deal with the maternal metabolites of any drugs, in addition to the drug itself. Large molecular weight drugs can block the passage of oxygen through the placental membrane and result in smaller babies (this is true also for smoked drugs, including nicotine).

Unless properly treated, fetal withdrawal symphoms from opiates can result in convulsions with consequent risk of brain damage or death. One of the problems with heavy drug use will be that the woman may neglect her nutritional needs and her physical health will suffer as a result. It is therefore the indirect lifestyle effect of drug use that may cause many of the observed problems in the infant, such as premature birth and low birth weight. Poor ante-natal care as a result of irregular attendance or attending late in pregnancy are further behavioural factors which can contribute to a higher incidence of obstetric complications for the mother, and a higher incidence of neonatal infections in the child.

Heroin

Of all psychotropic drugs, heroin has received most attention in terms of its effect on the fetus and its associated withdrawal syndrome in the infant. Due to its low molecular weight, heroin easily crosses the placental barrien.[9] Some studies have demonstrated low birth weight and premature delivery associated with heroin use during pregnancy.[10,11,12]

Withdrawal can cause strong fetal movements which increase oxygen consumption, and this can lead to lack of oxygen and possible death. There are a wide range of symptoms, the major signs of withdrawal in infants are:

- irritability, restlessness, twitchiness, shrill, high-pitched cry, seizures, sneezing, cramps;
- sleep disturbance;
- feed disturbance – increased or decreased milk intake, vomiting or diarrhoea;
- fever – sweaty, rapid heart rate, rapid breathing.

Seizures and feed disturbances, if severe, can lead to death if untreated and even sometimes when they are treated. The signs of fever can be confused as signs of infection which may complicate accurate diagnosis. There is only equivocal evidence for the long-term effects of heroin use on the infant. Minor motor disturbances and poor attention span have been found in children one year later.[13] The long-term effects of slowness in speech, and of language disorders, are unclear.[14]

These problems are more likely to be related to or associated with social disadvantages such as poor accommodation and nutritional neglect.

Prescribing during pregnancy

It is highly desirable that the pregnant woman talks to her worker about her drug use. This is much more likely to happen if the woman is reassured that she will not be discriminated against as a result of her drug use/HIV status; that she is not automatically going to have her baby taken away from her and that the service she receives will be understanding of her lifestyle/drug use. It is beneficial to both mother and baby that the woman be prescribed a substitute medication during her pregnancy as quickly as possible and with the minimum of preliminaries. In practice, methadone tends to be the substitute medication offered. Prescribing treatment for the woman can help stabilise her lifestyle with an attendant improvement in ante-natal attendance. Methadone has benefits for the unborn baby since it has been shown to decrease fetal wastage and improve interuterine growth.[15] This is more likely to be due to an indirect effect of stabilisation of the mother's lifestyle, more regular contact with health care services, and regular eating plus a clean drug supply. It also means that the staff know (roughly) what drugs are being used, and the severity of the infant's withdrawals can be approximately estimated.

According to Williams,[16] pregnant women attending prescribing drug services can be divided into two distinct groups:

(1) Those who became pregnant whilst on a methadone prescription.
(2) Those who commence a programme because they are pregnant.

The woman who belongs in group 1 is already established in a counselling relationship. She is more likely to register earlier on in the pregnancy for ante-natal care. She will be 'au fait' with the drug clinic regime. The woman from group 2 may be unfamiliar with the clinic system and the programme demands. She may not have had any desire to seek treatment were it not for the fact that she became pregnant. According to Williams, the IDU woman, on the one hand, 'must now comply with a somewhat arbitrary infantalising system and, on the other, must be prepared to accept responsibility for another human being'.

In either situation it is essential to establish that the prescribed medication is adequate for stabilisation of the woman's drug use, and that she can be open with you about this. Topping up when on a prescription will be common during pregnancy, perhaps not surprisingly since this is a period of greater stress and concern for the pregnant woman.

It should be possible for the woman to discuss increases in the methadone if she feels tempted to use other drugs or if urine screening indicates that she is topping up on a regular basis. Sometimes an increase in methadone is required during the third trimester of pregnancy due to tissue binding and metabolism of the drug.[17]

If the woman wants to withdraw totally or at least reduce to a minimum dosage (5–10 ml methadone per day), before her baby is born, then there is some controversy about how this should be done. Some argue that the reduction schedule should be gradual, 2–5 ml every 3/4 days, and should not take place during the first and third trimester due to the risk of miscarriage or premature delivery.[18] Others suggest 5 mg per week.[19,20] Still others suggest 5 mgs every other week between the 14th and 28th week of gestation.

Dosage reductions should, in principle, not be undertaken during the first trimester and not after the 32nd week of pregnancy. Increased rates of abortion have been reported during the first trimester and in the third trimester, as well as the occurrence of premature labour and sudden intrauterine death of the child.[18,21,22,23] However, a number of doctors have put women on much more rapid reduction schedules with no adverse effects at all. Whatever reduction schedule is agreed, it is important that the woman feels that she has some control over this. Small decreases indicate she is making an effort and should be encouraged.

A number of reports indicate that the incidence of complications in mothers and children who have been in a methadone withdrawal programme corresponds with the rate of complications in a 'normal' population.[24,25,26,27] Methadone-maintained women spend less time in hospital than the heroin user.[14] If the woman has reduced to 10–15 ml methadone before giving birth, then the infant may not go into withdrawal or at least show only minimal signs. Reduction of methadone may be encouraged by some obstetricians and midwives. The drug worker may not feel this is appropriate, particularly if the woman has been stable on a maintenance prescription prior to her pregnancy. After her ante-natal appointment, Jan called her drug worker and said, 'I'm really frightened, I rely on my methadone to keep me straight; they said I have to come off'. She had to be reassured that she would not be reduced against her will. This was reinforced by subsequent liaison with her midwife. Detoxification the first year after the birth may be more suitable if things are going well for mother and child and she is still stable. Appropriate care during pregnancy can have far reaching implications for future drug use.

Infant withdrawal

The drugs used to control infant withdrawal will vary from hospital to hospital and range from chlorpromazine (Largactil), morphine, methadone, diazepam, phenobarbitone, clonidine, Lomotil and Phenergan. The drugs used to control withdrawal may themselves cause problems, chlorpromazine, for example, can make the baby become drowsy and lethargic and this results in poor sucking reflex and consequent lack of weight gain. It is difficult to predict the duration of heroin withdrawal for the baby, but this may last for about a week after birth. Because of the variable strength of illicit heroin, the fetus can face the risk not only of withdrawal but also of maternal overdose. If the woman suddenly stops taking heroin, the damage can occur in the fetus before the mother becomes aware that she is beginning to suffer from withdrawals. Tylden and Finnegan[18,28] reported cases of fetal death after sudden heroin withdrawal during pregnancy.

Methadone withdrawal may last considerably longer than heroin withdrawal (up to three months, although this is very rare), and may not become apparent until two weeks after delivery, causing problems over the period of discharge of the baby from hospital. This can be extremely frustrating for the parents. Many paediatricians prefer not to use methadone as a substitute medication during pregnancy due to the problems it causes for the newborn baby in terms of drug withdrawal. It lasts longer in the baby's system due to its longer half-life and can produce more severe and prolonged drug withdrawal for the baby than heroin.

Respiratory distress is said to be higher in children of methadone-substituted mothers.[29] Glass *et al.*[30] observed no cases of respiratory distress syndrome among children of heroin-dependent mothers born between the 32nd and 37th week of pregnancy. The frequency of fits in children on methadone-substituted mothers is also said to be higher.[23] The effects of other drugs on the fetus have not been extensively documented.

Cocaine and crack

Cocaine use constricts blood vessels and as a result of this blood flow to the fetus is restricted. This drug has been implicated in an increased incidence of stillbirths, separation from the placenta, and spontaneous abortions.[31] A relationship has also been suggested between cocaine use and gastrointestinal birth defects in the neonate.[32] The withdrawal syndrome in the infant is characterised by irritability, poor feeding and difficulty in being comforted. If withdrawal symptoms are observed they will usually require the infant to be kept in hospital for a couple of weeks.

Amphetamines

An indirect effect of amphetamine use is that the woman may neglect her diet. As a result of poor diet she may be unable to sustain the nutritional needs of the fetus. Amphetamine use leads to difficulty in the absorption of calcium, therefore the woman can experience lots of cramps during the pregnancy and suffer from weakened bones and teeth. The baby may be small. There has been a suggested association between amphetamine use, heart problems and cleft palate abnormalities in the infant.[18]

Barbiturates

Barbiturate use has been associated with congenital abnormalities in the infant.[18] It can also lead to withdrawal effects in the fetus in the later stages of pregnancy.

Benzodiazepines

These very widely used drugs can cause withdrawal symptoms in the fetus, especially if large doses have been taken regularly during the pregnancy. According to Tylden,[18] passive withdrawal can develop in a fetus whose mother has been using these drugs.

Cannabis

There have been some suggestions that cannabis use is associated with premature birth, but there is no firm evidence for this. However, smoking may cause problems since it interferes with absorption across the placenta.

Glue and solvent sniffing

Solvent use has been associated with smallness in the fetus and congenital abnormalities.

Alcohol

The fetal alcohol syndrome as a result of alcohol use during pregnancy has been well documented. It causes a characteristic pattern of developmental and psychological problems in the infant.

Counselling the drug-using woman during pregnancy

For a drug-using woman with low self esteem, having a child can seem like the one worthwhile thing she can do. The desire to have a baby can vary between the overt 'we're trying to get pregnant', to 'if it happened I'd quite like it'. In others the desire for a child is a desperate need. As a result of being HIV-positive, many IDUs have a sense of urgency added to their desire for a child. Having children (provided you are able to take care of them physically, emotionally and materially) is something that is respected in our society.

One client was quite struck by the positive attention she received from 'straight' people when she was out with her baby, people who, previously, she felt completely alienated from. The desire for a baby can be a much more urgent issue for the drug user who is faced with a life-threatening condition. There is a strong desire to have a baby and, perhaps for continuity, to leave something of yourself behind. The hope that the child will be unaffected by HIV is frequently reinforced by knowing someone else with HIV whose baby was OK. Idealised views prevail.

Unfortunately, there are also many problems for the drug using parent. Having idealised parenthood, they may have an unrealistic outlook about how they are going to cope as parents. Frequently they have to work with an increased number of professionals concerned with the baby's care; in addition, they will have to cope with their drug problem as well as the demands the baby makes on their time, often in conditions of socio-economic deprivation. Basically, the odds are stacked against them. Practical needs are paramount. In one study, an established residence corresponded to a greater degree of parenting among drug-using women than did participation in methadone treatment or prenatal care.[13]

If the woman's partner is a drug user, he may not be able to support the woman due to his own drug use. Being a single parent is tough enough, but being a single parent with a drug problem is doubly difficult. Bashore *et al.*[33] found that pregnant heroin users were younger than non-addicted pregnant women and more likely to be separated or divorced from their partner.

In contrast to the reality of their lives, most drug-dependent women hold very conservative views of women as wives and mothers.[16] The contrast between what they believe a good mother is and what they are able to be makes these women extremely vulnerable to low self esteem and guilt. Problems can begin to emerge within the first year and especially when the baby starts to run around and become more demanding. There is often a fear that they will lose their children, although the Advisory Council on the Misuse of Drugs has recommended that drug use in itself should not constitute grounds for placing the baby on the 'at risk' register. Local authority policy in terms of interpretation of the risks to the child as a result of parental drug use will vary from place to place.

Despite the problems, pregnancy can be a powerful learning experience for the woman in terms of exerting some control over her drug use. In Edinburgh HIV-positive women with no pregnancies have been found to have a higher incidence of continued drug use than those with pregnancies among whom drug use had been reduced.[34] Fried *et al.*[35] found a hang-over influence of the control exerted during pregnancy in terms of reduced soft drug use (nicotine, alcohol and cannabis) one year later. So pregnancy and the control the client may achieve during pregnancy can be an important learning experience. Pregnancy may also be a time when the client is much more likely to want to (or at least consider) planning ahead.

HIV counselling during pregnancy

Information about pregnancy and HIV can be one of the most difficult areas on which to give counsel. This is due both to the emotive nature of the subject and the ever changing statistics on transmission risk to the child. It is striking how long it took for updated information on pregnancy to become incorporated into the counselling that staff gave to clients. There is also the problem that clients themselves have in 'hearing' information when it is not the advice they want. Sophie, for example, an HIV-positive IDU, protested angrily after hearing the latest statistics, 'that I just did not want her to have a baby, no one did'. It emerged that she had been to at least four different professionals for information, none of whom had said she should not have children, but simply gave her the up-to-date information on transmission. She had wanted someone to tell her there was no risk; she could not find someone to do this and therefore interpreted us as trying to put her off.

Sometimes the client expresses concern about people's reactions if they know the woman is HIV-positive and pregnant. Gill's is a case in point. Most of the people on the housing estate where she lived, knew about Gill being HIV-positive. This was because she and her partner had got drunk and had a loud argument on their doorstep about her having AIDS. She had been subjected to verbal and physical harassment from her neighbours as a result. While waiting for a housing transfer, she became pregnant and told her worker that she was scared about what would happen, 'when she started to show'. 'They're bad enough now, but if they see I'm going to have a baby, what with the AIDS and all, I don't know what they'll be like.'

Ante-natal HIV screening

HIV antibody testing in pregnancy has been recommended for the following reasons:

(1) The woman can make an informed choice about whether or not she wishes to become pregnant or, if already pregnant, continue with the pregnancy.
(2) The woman can be offered medical supervision and treatment.
(3) The baby can be appropriately monitored and treated.[36]

The above is much more likely to happen if the woman is reassured that she will not be discriminated against as a result of being HIV-antibody-positive. Screening programmes that seek to identify 'high risk' people are unlikely to work. Screening is of benefit to clients only if they can make an informed choice and if management of HIV is available to them. Ryder[37] found that seropositive women who were detected during an ante-natal screening programme became pregnant again soon after learning their result. The role of the ante-natal clinic in testing for HIV is controversial. Wherever testing is carried out, there should be adequate opportunity for pre- and post-test counselling and this is not always practical in some ante-natal settings.

Effect of pregnancy on health of HIV-positive women

Pregnancy causes immune suppression. It has therefore been suggested that the cumulative effect of HIV infection and pregnancy might accelerate the progression of HIV disease in women.

The effect of pregnancy on a mother's health seems to depend on the stage of HIV disease that she has reached. In basic terms, the advice is the earlier the better – in stages II and III of HIV infection, the woman's health is unaffected. In stage IV, where there may be clear evidence of damage to the woman's immune system, then her health may be adversely affected by pregnancy and, if infected, the outcome for the child may be worse. Therefore, avoidance of pregnancy at this stage may be advisable. Apart from the symptoms and signs that the woman will have at stage IV, certain blood tests will help clarify her prognosis. However, there is no clear evidence as yet that pregnancy worsens maternal prognosis as measured by laboratory tests or clinical disease progression.[38] In a three-year follow-up of age-matched HIV-positive pregnant versus HIV-positive non-pregnant women, no difference was found between the two groups at three-year follow-up in terms of the clinical stage of the disease, T4 counts, and other laboratory tests.[39]

In another study which compared HIV-positive and -negative pregnant women, all women (positive and negative) were found to have reduced T4 counts during pregnancy. The positive women had a greater fall of T4 cells during pregnancy and this was sustained after the birth. It was concluded that although no clinical evidence exists for HIV disease worsening in those women who become pregnant whilst at CDCII and III, pregnancy might worsen T-cell function.

Based on a three-year follow-up study in Edinburgh, HIV disease progression has been shown to be associated with increasing age of seroconversion. Injecting drug use in itself did not appear to independently worsen prognosis.[40] Of 218 women studied in Edinburgh, the researchers were unable to demonstrate an adverse effect due to pregnancy.

HIV transmission from mother to baby

According to the current findings of the European collaborative study on HIV and pregnancy, there is a 13% risk of transmission from mother to baby.[41] Of those children who are infected, 83% show laboratory or clinical signs of infection by six months of age. By 12 months, 26% have AIDS and 17% die of HIV-related disease. This figure has undergone a number of revisions as the opportunity for longitudinal research has developed.

Route of transmission from mother to baby

During pregnancy

The likely route of transmission is across the placenta. HIV has been found in fetal tissue as early as 15 weeks into pregnancy. The virus has also been grown *in vitro* in amniotic fluid and placental tissue.

During delivery

The effect of exposure to HIV during delivery is equivocal. Isolation of virus from amniotic and vaginal secretions – as well as obvious exposure to maternal blood during vaginal delivery or caesarean section – make this mode of transmission plausible.

In a study carried out in twins and triplets born to women infected with the virus, Goedert *et al.* found that although some infants may be infected *in utero*, a substantial proportion of firstborns became infected as they came into contact with the cervix and birth canal.[42]

Care and pain relief in pregnancy and during birth

Many types of professionals will be involved with the parents' and child's care; this can be beneficial for the client but sometimes it leads to duplication of work. Like HIV, pregnancy makes workers want to react. Social workers have a statutory responsibility to do so. A combination of the two, however, can leave the client in the background whilst the workers try to 'help'. Liaison at all stages is essential. There is a danger of overhelping, especially when the client dumps the same problems on different staff. With the mother's help, however, some very fruitful co-operation effort can emerge. The worker needs to be realistic about what can be achieved by both themselves and the client. They should also be prepared to set boundaries: being able to say 'no', for instance, when the client wants inappropriate things. Sophie, for example, was not pregnant. She was trying to have a baby and had a worker in the syringe exchange, the home support team, the DDU, and also had regular contact with the STD clinic doctor. She then wanted a midwife as well.

There will always be clients who refuse assistance although you know they would benefit from involvement with your agency. Conversely, there may be instances when workers have to intervene when clients refuse assistance.

If you are working with a pregnant drug user, it can be helpful to arm yourself with the following facts about your own unit:

- where does your responsibility lie? Most of the recent child-related guidelines say that all agencies in contact with children have a responsibility to develop a child-centred focus;
- does your unit have a policy about working with parents and children? Is this made available to clients?
- do you have clear reporting procedures if you are concerned about the welfare of the child? Are the parents aware of your role in this referral process?
- is your unit 'child friendly', i.e. a safe environment, with pushchair access, toys, clothes?
- is the pregnant user on prescribed medication? If not, are you in a position to do anything about this?
- if the pregnant user *is* on prescribed medication, is this adequate for stabilisation of the drug problem? Can the woman be open with you about this issue?
- are multi-agency/team meetings possible for workers involved in the client's care?
- do the parents have access, if they want it, to adequate support and counselling to discuss their anxieties about the well-being of the child?
- are you providing accurate, up-to-date information on HIV transmission in pregnancy?

In addition, it is useful for the worker to inform themselves with the facts about other services as follows:

- which other professionals are you able/unable to discuss the case with, i.e. GP, health visitor, etc.;
- do the parents have access to adequate welfare and benefits?
- is the housing situation suitable for parents and child? If not, are you in a position to do anything about this?
- can you ensure that ante-natal appointments are at realistic times of the day and do not clash with other appointments, such as drug dependency clinic? If on the same site, can these appointments be co-ordinated for the same day? Could prescribing be organised from the ante-natal clinic?
- do the parents want you to introduce them to the ante-natal and other staff who will be involved in their care, and vice versa?
- can the paediatrician be introduced to the parents before the birth of the child?
- what is the policy of the ante-natal clinic with respect to HIV-antibody testing?
- is it possible for mother and baby to stay together on the post-natal ward while the baby is under observation for drug withdrawal?
- is it possible for paediatric follow-up appointments to be community-based (as, for example, in Edinburgh)?
- are you aware of local fostering/adoption facilities? Is respite care available if the parents require it?
- is there access to a residential facility that can care for the pregnant woman, mother or parents and the baby if residential detoxification is desired?
- is specialist termination counselling available?
- is there access to termination facilities if the mother wants this?
- What is the policy regarding infection control, i.e. do they expect to be informed of the woman's HIV status and are you prepared/unprepared to co-operate with this?

According to Williams,[16] it is also useful for the worker to provide the following information:

- explanations of the course of pregnancy;
- information about the ante-natal clinic and waiting times. Explanations of ante-natal procedures and care, e.g. the recognition and care of the infant's withdrawal syndrome and the difficulty in predicting the duration of this. This may be provided by organised groups in

the drug clinic with invited speakers from ante-natal services;
- the policy of the ante-natal clinic on antibody testing;
- explanations to the client about the way ante-natal services work. The drug worker can enable the client to be assertive in their response to ante-natal staff rather than developing the passive/aggressive style which some women adopt. This can be achieved by role playing and modelling the appropriate behaviours.

Often the client almost expects to be treated badly and their own painful feelings can be masked by anger, hostility and sometimes challenging behaviour. The IDU can be extremely sensitive to slights or negative attitudes. The drug worker, understanding this, can act as an interpreter in angry, hostile or otherwise inexplicable behaviour to other staff.

If possible the drug worker should make him- or herself known to the hospital or ante-natal clinic and needs to have an awareness of the practices and conduct at these facilities so that they can make a realistic contribution. Obviously this is more difficult for them if they are short staffed and geographically removed. Some workers attend initial appointments with their client. Even telephone contact, with the client's consent, may help. The drug workers' experience needs to be taken into account by other staff; they should not be considered to be merely watchdogs for missed appointments and the monitoring of drug use through urine tests.

Pain relief in labour

A major concern is the type and level of analgesic drugs given during labour. Pain thresholds are often very low and tolerance to analgesics is very high. Making the woman aware that her particular situation will be taken into consideration can help enormously, i.e. telling her before she goes into labour what drugs will be given and to what levels. Find out the levels she thinks she might need. The importance of finding out exactly what the woman has used can be emphasised to her; there may, for example, be a risk of overdose if the woman has been using opiates beforehand and opiate pain relief is administered. Epidurals will be effective. A very high proportion of births to drug-using women are by caesarean section.[36] It would be interesting to determine whether the reason for this is related to lowered pain thresholds and pain management during labour.

Infection control

This is one of the most important places for a 'one tier' (i.e. non-segregating) infection control policy where adequate staff safety precautions are taken in the labour room for *every* woman who uses the service. This ensures that the HIV-positive woman is not singled out or treated as different from everyone else. No one maternity unit should have to be singled out to specialise in these deliveries, since this serves to alienate those who have HIV infection and also leads to a false sense of security in the non-specialist units.

The risk of contact with blood and other body fluids plus risk of needlestick injury is high in the delivery room. In 202 vaginal deliveries and 29 caesarean sections involving health care workers, 118 blood contacts and 38 amniotic fluid contacts occurred. Although seroconversion rates following needlestick injury are low, it is important to minimise the risks wherever possible. In the delivery room this involves the appropriate use of disposable or sterilisable equipment such as gloves, spectacles, waterproof gowns, and avoiding re-sheathing used needles. Staff compliance will depend on factors such as loss of manual dexterity as a result of the thickness of the gloves and lack of time due to emergencies. There is also an attitudinal component since some workers feel that it puts barriers between them and the mother and is an unacceptable medicalisation of labour. Where possible, all health care workers and counselling staff should have hepatitis B vaccination.

Even if you work in a non-medical setting, infection control procedures for dealing with body fluid spillages need to be clarified. This was brought home to me the day a pregnant client was sick in my waste paper basket! We had another incident where the client squeezed blood and pus from an abscess on her hand in and around the sink in the office while she waited for the doctor to come and attend to her. Adequate facilities for safe disposal and incineration of syringes is thus likely to be required. There should be a ready supply of disposable gloves, disinfectants, etc.

If exposure should occur, via a needlestick injury, for example, the site should be squeezed to encourage bleeding, cleaned, and bandaged. AZT has been given to health care workers in some cases where possible exposure to HIV has occurred. To be of any benefit in prevention of infection, AZT should be taken within 24 hours (preferably within one hour). Access to counselling may also be required.

Post-natal care

The parents must be prepared for the treatment their baby will receive if it has to go into Special Care, babies in withdrawal, for example, may be set off from the main unit. Some mothers may interpret this as seeking to hide or reject their babies. One HIV-positive client described her care when two years previously she had given birth to a baby boy. She was kept in a side room with a warning notice on the door. Any staff who came near her (even to give her meals) wore gloves and masks. Whilst waiting in her room to leave the hospital with her baby she watched a member of staff come in, dispose of her sheets, and begin to wash the bed down with disinfectant. Nothing was explained to her and, two years later, she was still unable to talk about the experience without breaking down because of the shame and isolation she had experienced. It only takes one member of staff with a biased, negative attitude to ruin all of the good work of those who go before them.

Ideally, the mother should be with the baby as much as possible, but limited resources may mean that she is unable to stay over at the hospital. The parents' own behaviour may reduce the chances of this happening: time spent scoring drugs – and the effect of the drugs themselves – may mean that they do not make the visits at appropriate times; one father, for example, regularly used to turn up to see his son at 3 am.

'When my baby was born she had a high pitched cry and I remember thinking "how sweet". I now know that this is a sign of my baby being addicted.' (An ex-drug-user.) Although it can be very difficult to do at times, if the parent(s) can be involved as much as possible then this can be very helpful: they should, for example, be aware of the drugs being used for withdrawal and the dosage regime.

It is also helpful if the mother can be kept with her child in order, along with the specialist nursing staff, to help with observation of signs of withdrawal. (The mechanics of this will depend on ward policy and staffing levels.) When babies do require care in neonatal units they can be very demanding of the staff's attention; they may cry for long periods of time and respond only to swaddling and cuddling. Two or three of these babies in a unit together can make enormous demands on staff time; 'cuddling' often gets left to the more junior, less experienced staff. In the USA there are teams of volunteers in some hospitals who come onto the neonatal care units specifically to cuddle and rock these babies. It can be very difficult for staff, particularly if they have no training regarding drug use, the drug user's lifestyle, and how drug treatment facilities operate. Liaison with parents can be difficult as the staff are often required to observe parent/child interaction for the post-birth care conference and parents may resent this. When monitoring mother–baby behaviour, staff should explain this and involve the parents. Make sure that they remind staff to make a note of their visits, encourage telephone contact if they cannot visit, ensure awareness of night shift visits. In this way, both mother and father get credit for their involvement in the baby's care.

Parents' guilt feelings about the effect of their drug use on the baby may be translated into 'difficult' interactions with the staff. The staff may have problems caring for the baby who is so obviously adversely affected by the parents' drug use. They may experience distress as they anticipate what the baby is going out to. It is necessary to allow the staff the opportunity to express these feelings and, more generally, around the deaths that may occur among the babies in their care. They may be assisted to come to a better understanding of the issues in one-to-one support or in regular facilitated support groups preferably with a facilitator with some experience of drug work and/or bereavement.

'When my baby was in the special care unit, I had the feeling that I was being kept at arms length by the staff. I felt very isolated and terribly guilty. My drug use had increased. If someone could have reached out, if I had felt there was a friendly face, it would have made all the difference.' Seeing other mothers with their families can emphasise the IDUs feelings of isolation. An important factor is that the neonatal staff may have access to clients when they are vulnerable and perhaps receptive to advice and information. In order to make constructive use of this situation it is desirable that staff are familiar with drug issues as well as harm minimisation, local treatment facilities, syringe exchange and family planning services.

Sometimes the parents' guilt and feelings of anxiety for their child can be translated into exaggerated concern. Elaine, for example, took her baby to Accident and Emergency at 1 am because he had nappy rash. She frequently misses her appointments with the paediatrician because she is frightened that he will tell her that her baby has seroconverted. What is usually a time of pleasure for the parents and relatives can become a nightmare if the child's parents want to keep their worries for their child to themselves. 'I was almost afraid to tell them (her parents) I'd had Sheila. I was so wound up and scared I just kept bursting into tears. I knew they wouldn't understand and would start asking questions.' The worker can encourage the child's parents to take their time and not to rush into involving other family members until they feel ready to cope with their reactions.

Confidentiality

'When my baby was in special care, other mothers used to ask me what was wrong with her. At first I didn't know what to say, then I told them it was diabetes.' It can be extremely difficult to maintain confidentiality under the circumstances that exist on the post-natal ward and special care unit. If the parents are concerned then staff can help by being careful about discussing the baby's care in areas where other mothers can hear. Perhaps going along with an 'acceptable' explanation for why the baby is in the unit.

IDUs can be sensitive to being treated in any way different from other parents. At the same time, they may be insecure about mixing with other mothers and therefore avoid going to where they would have to meet them, to parentcraft classes, for example. Mary, an HIV-positive woman, was convinced that she would be kept in a room on her own. She threatened to go somewhere else where they did not know her if this turned out to be true. It must never be forgotten that the woman has the right to 'vote with her feet' and go elsewhere. Coercion and judgmental treatment will increase the risk of this happening. Mary's anxieties were eased enormously when she was taken on a tour of the maternity unit by her midwife with whom she had developed a strong, trusting relationship. The midwife had made it quite clear to Mary that her ante-natal welfare was her first concern and other professionals (such as drug workers) were concerned with other aspects of her care. This made a vast difference to her receptiveness to ante-natal care and facilitated bonding with her baby.

Breast feeding

HIV has been found in breast milk. Eight cases have been reported where transmission via breast feeding was implicated as the route of transmission. There have been cases of mothers known not to be infected at the time of delivery who, during the immediate post partum period (usually through receipt of HIV-infected blood transfusion), became infected with HIV. There was also one case where the wet nurse was found to be HIV-positive.

In all these cases, all but one of the women were at a stage of HIV where the virus was active and therefore possible present at higher concentrations in body fluids. Furthermore, the relatively small number of (eight) cases does not really constitute an adequate number from which to draw firm conclusions. Although they define a risk they fail to provide insight into the importance of breast milk as a transmission vehicle. No information is available from these cases on the concentration of the virus in milk, the presence of neutralising antibodies, or the woman's level of immunodeficiency.

In the UK, HIV-positive women have been advised not to breastfeed (Department of Health guidelines), and not to contribute to milk banks.[43] In countries where resources are low, funding is not always available to offer substitutes for breast milk. Breast milk confers immunity to other diseases for children and is therefore very important. Even in developed countries, breastfeeding has been shown to have noticeably beneficial effect on children's health in comparison to those who are not breastfed. A recent study in Glasgow showed the benefits of breast feeding for babies in a large city.[44] Breastfeeding will also be important where the child may be of low birth weight due to the mother's poor nutritional state as a result of drug use. The psychological and emotional benefits to the mother are also well documented. Whether or not the woman is symptomatic at the time of delivery will be relevant, but there have not yet been any prospective studies, and the ultimate decision should rest with the mother.

One HIV-positive woman keep coming to the ward sister with suggestions about how to make her milk safe for her baby: 'what if I express it, and then have it pasteurised?' She was very disturbed that she could not breastfeed her child. Other clients will not even entertain the idea due to the potential risk. A major obstacle to the IDU woman is not the small amount of methadone in her milk, but the prolonged separation of mother and child if the baby is withdrawing from drugs. Demand feeding is difficult, so is establishing and maintaining a milk supply. It can involve frequent hospital visits and use of a breast pump at home. This is a major investment of time and energy. Too vigorous promotion of breastfeeding may develop a sense of inadequacy and failure in the mother. The stability of the mother's drug use may be another factor to take into consideration. If the mother continues to use drugs such as cocaine and then breastfeeds, this can be a problem for her continued drug use as the effects of the drug will rapidly become apparent in the baby. Prescribed methadone will not pose a significant difficulty, but if quantities of illicit drugs are being used as well, then it may adversely affect the baby. Amanda: 'I really wanted to breastfeed. That night I used a lot of cocaine. I remember she fed well, but later on she convulsed. I stopped breastfeeding; she had become a threat to my drug use. When I think about that now, it makes me very sad.'

Isolated evidence of mothers being infected by their babies has been reported in what was the USSR.[45] Eight women contracted HIV through breastfeeding their babies (who had been infected by re-use of contaminated needles and syringes). No other risk factors were known for these women. In each case, the children had bleeding from the mouth from candida infection; blood from the babies' mouths entered the mothers' bloodstream through cracks in the women's nipples. This constitutes a rare form of blood-to-blood transmission.

Assessing a child's HIV status

Once a baby is born to a mother with HIV it can take up to 18 months before the HIV status of the baby can be accurately determined. This is because babies will be born with their mother's antibodies. Therefore, a positive HIV-antibody test result on a baby performed before this time has elapsed will reveal the mother's antibody status. After an average of 18 months, the mother's antibodies will usually have disappeared and an HIV-antibody test at this stage will give a more reliable picture of the baby's antibody status. It is unlikely that an antibody test will in itself be considered sufficient confirmation of the baby's status. Other blood tests and examinations will probably be carried out before this 'waiting time' has elapsed. There are, however, often procedural and interpretational difficulties with many of these tests.

Antigen test (p24)

This test involves identification of certain HIV-related proteins. In a study carried out in New York, 66% of children less than six months old who were HIV-seropositive were also p24 antigen positive.[46] Antigen-positive children have been shown to have a worse prognosis than similarly aged seropositive children who were antigen-negative.[47] The disadvantage of this test is that it has not been fully evaluated and also requires a quantity of serum difficult to obtain from each infant.

Blood culture

This involves attempting to cultivate the virus under laboratory conditions. This can be difficult to do so a negative result does not necessarily mean that the virus is not present. According to Mok,[48] 50 ml of blood is required for this test to be carried out on an adult.

From infants she takes only 1–5 ml. The sensitivity of the test is thus diminished by at least five-fold.

Immunoglobulin testing

A specific immune response of the infant that would indicate infection is the presence of IgG, IgA or IgM antibodies. These antibodies do not cross the placenta. According to Wieblen[49] this is an effective method for early diagnosis of HIV-infected infants who have no other signs of infection. In the European collaborative study, without a definitive virological diagnosis, the monitoring of immunoglobulins, CD4/CD8 ratio, and clinical signs could identify infection in 48% of infected children by six months with a specificity of more than 99%.[41]

Polymerase chain reaction (PCR)

Diagnosis of HIV infection in babies is now more accurate because of this test. This is a highly sensitive DNA detection method. Sequences of DNA are amplified over a million times in a few hours. With automation, PCR is likely to provide the diagnostic sensitivity which inhibits the current efforts to determine the incidence of perinatal infection. Although it is a very sensitive method, due to its high cost and susceptibility to environmental contamination, it is still regarded as a research tool. Some children do not make HIV-specific antibodies.[37,50] There are a number of reports of antibody-negative children with AIDS.[50,51] Inability to mount a classic immunological response to infection probably derives from the stage of their HIV infection and the damage caused to their immune systems. PCR-sensitive antigen detection or viral cultures will enable these children to be properly diagnosed. Until these tests become more widely used, parents have to cope with chronic anxiety about the health of their child. The impact of this should not be underestimated.

Termination of pregnancy

The decision of whether or not to terminate a pregnancy will depend on whether the woman wants the baby, not on the basis of HIV.[52,53] Inability to accurately diagnose HIV infection in the unborn child is also likely to be an important factor. The vast majority of women requesting termination of pregnancy do so for social reasons and not because of HIV seropositivity.[52]

The decision to terminate should be the woman's decision. Often she 'knows someone' who has had children with HIV and they were fine. However, this experience is frequently based on women who were asymptomatic or at least had not yet developed severe illness.

As well as her state of health at the time, other influences will be the health prospects of the child, the stage of pregnancy at the time of presentation, and the psychological, social and practical support that is available.

Being anti-abortion is another factor that will influence the woman not to have a termination of pregnancy. If the woman does decide to have her pregnancy terminated, however, it is much better done in early pregnancy. Because of the frequent late presentation of drug users, there is the added risk that the pregnancy is sometimes well advanced before the decision is reached. This can necessitate urgent access to termination of pregnancy services. It is therefore essential that these links are established before they are required. There should be a pre-existing procedure for access to a termination service if the woman wants this. Access to specialist abortion counsellors can be very useful, both in terms of facilitating the woman's decision and in going through the pros and cons, preparation for the abortion, and how she will cope afterwards. The counsellor can help the woman by explaining some of the conflicting emotions she may experience: relief, for example, that she is no longer pregnant versus grief for the loss of someone she will never know. Some women who have had terminations report 'wondering' about this for years later: 'he/she would be 12 by now', 'I wonder what he/she would have looked like.' Abortion is often a hidden loss, and women may not have told anyone else about it. It is therefore important to have someone who will be able to acknowledge her feelings.

Miscarriages and still births will also give rise to feelings of grief and loss. Many maternity units will offer parents the option of seeing or holding their dead baby and may indeed encourage this in order that the loss is validated and becomes tangible. Longer term support may be necessary.

Prophylactic care in pregnancy

Knowledge of the effects of AZT during pregnancy are limited. Treatment regimes are therefore uncertain. The question for those who are on this drug when they become pregnant is whether to stop it in pregnancy or not. It may be that continuing on it improves maternal and fetal prognosis by reducing quantity of virus in the mother and therefore the rate of vertical transmission. AZT crosses the placenta and its presence in fetal blood may also prevent infection. However, the potential side effects (particularly long-term) to the fetus are unknown. The dilemma is that if it is stopped during pregnancy then maternal prognosis may worsen. Studies are under way to assess whether AZT administered during labour may reduce maternal transmission. After the birth one problem that can arise is trying to get the mother to take care of her own health, especially with respect to medication like AZT. Frequently the woman's health seems to take second place to concern for her child's health.

Case study of Josie

Finally, it is hoped that the following case study will help illustrate some of the points being made in this chapter.

Josie was a HIV-positive woman known to the drug worker for two years prior to her pregnancy. She was tested elsewhere. She was always extremely anxious on contact with the DDU. She never stayed long and very rarely attended appointments on time. She often dropped out of treatment and came back expecting to be put on a prescription immediately. She became angry and tearful if she had to wait. Contact with her was nearly always characterised by crisis. There was no opportunity to discuss safer sex or injecting. She had poor injecting technique, poor veins, and lots of scar tissue from abscesses that she had not had properly treated. She never disclosed using on top of her prescription, but eventually the worker was able to introduce her to the syringe exchange service which she started to use regularly.

Josie's pregnancy was confirmed in the DDU using a Ramp pregnancy test provided by the family planning doctor. This test gives a result in about two minutes. A midwife who was very committed to good standards of care for IDUs was contacted and came to the DDU to see her. Josie was very anxious but, after an initial session, the midwife booked her in and was able to get a junior doctor to meet her at the DDU and then take her (accompanied by her drug worker) to the clinic for examination and tests. Josie had a chronic fear that her baby would be taken from her. Other users would wind her up about the baby being taken away and then she would come to the DDU and threaten to go somewhere else where she was not known to have her baby. She had to be continuously reassured.

Josie's partner did not know about her HIV status and she would not countenance telling him, stating that he had had a previous relationship with a girl who had died of AIDS. Josie asked that her drug worker stay with her during subsequent examinations at the ante-natal clinic and her syringe exchange worker stay with her at a number of others. She could not read or write and would not ask questions. She began to stabilise on her methadone and reduced her dosage without telling her worker. As trust developed she did disclose this and co-operated with regulating her dosage. Josie had had two previous children. Her mother took care of the first child. She deeply resented statutory services because when she became pregnant the second time, she wanted her baby to be adopted because she was 'strung out'. Her social worker had encouraged her to keep the child, but as a result of her drug use, the situation broke down and the child was removed.

She refused at first to see the social worker, but, eventually, she agreed to a brief accompanied visit. At first she refused to talk and left. But the next time she was more relaxed and reassured by the social worker. Eventually Josie saw her willingly on her own.

Josie managed to reduce to 5 ml methadone a day prior to the birth. During labour she wanted minimal pain relief. Due to liaison between midwife and neonatal staff, and a policy change on the unit, Josie was allowed to keep the baby with her and observations for withdrawal were carried out by Josie and the other nurses. The baby did not withdraw. The day after giving birth she asked for her prescription to be increased 'because she was afraid she might mess up'. This was arranged immediately. She bottlefed her baby who was able to go home with her on discharge. A planning meeting was organised in the absence of the midwife and drug worker, but due to her co-operative behaviour during the pregnancy, it was decided that she did not require further social services input.

After the brith she attended the DDU regularly and telephoned when she could not attend. She went through bouts of depression about her own and her baby's health and got very angry and upset with people for not telling her that her baby would be fine. She was on antidepressants for about a year after the birth. Josie still does not want to hear things that make her anxious, and mishears information about HIV. 'I thought you told me all babies are the same as mine; they are all born with the antibodies.' She is often frantic with worry over her baby. She does not understand her baby's paediatrician, so her drug worker telephones him to verify what has been said and goes over this information with her. He calls the drug worker when Josie misses appointments. Prescription collection is co-ordinated with these appointments. Messages can be left for her with her local pharmacist where she collects her methadone. She trusts her pharmacist; he understands her position and gives messages to her verbally. She shoplifts in order to keep her baby perfectly clothed which puts her at risk, but it is very important that she shows to the outside world what a good mother she is by dressing her baby well. Her partner still doesn't know about her HIV status. She continues to suffer from chronic anxiety over whether her baby will be OK. 'If anything happens to her, I'll kill myself.' Her baby has not yet cleared maternal antibodies, although blood cultures were negative. Josie continues to wait.

A number of points emerge from this case:

- the planning meeting (sometimes called the case conference) is a time of extreme anxiety and resentment and can leave parents feeling helpless and vulnerable. This can be greatly reduced if efforts are made to explain the procedure to them and involve them as far as possible, e.g. the legal process, the fact that there may be people there that they have not met before, the presence of the police;
- the behind the scenes liaison (with the client's consent) was time-consuming for all the workers involved, but it is necessary and worthwhile to allow sufficient time for this liaison to take place;
- a highly motivated midwife provided an essential liaison link. The client has better relationships with workers generally as a result of her experience;
- the prescribing policy was flexible and allowed her the space to stabilise her drug use. However, the prescribing of antidepressants may be perceived by some workers as treating the problem with more drugs – although this was on a short-term basis;
- waiting to establish the outcome for baby is a period of chronic anxiety. Josie still misses appointments.
- she has not accepted the implications of HIV for herself, or for the baby. Patience and tolerance is required on the worker's part.

One of the essential points that emerges from the above is that everyone (including drug workers), succeeded in adopting a mother–child focus, something which is not always the case.

HIV infection and AIDS in children

There are certain characteristic features of HIV infection and AIDS in children. The prognosis tends to be worse in children than in adults. There can be failure to thrive. They can also develop a more acute and severe form of *Pneumocystis carinii* pneumonia (PCP) than that seen in adults. Another frequent infection, seen only in children, is lymphoid interstitial pneumonitis, a chronic inflammation of lung tissue which causes breathing difficulties on exertion. Other non-specific bacterial infections can also be present which make a clear diagnosis difficult.

CDC HIV classification for children

The following classification system is that most commonly used:

(1) Indeterminate. Children less than 15 months who have been exposed, but who have not been antibody-tested (because the test is unhelpful).
(2) Children 'infected but asymptomatic', i.e. have no symptoms at all and are healthy carriers. Further subdivided as follows:
  (a) those with normal immune function;
  (b) those with abnormal immune function, i.e. low T-4 cell count.
(3) Symptomatic children. These are further subdivided as follows:
  (a) non-specific symptoms of early stages of disease: failure to thrive, PGL, unexplained fever, enlarged liver or spleen, persistent diarrhoea.
  (b) those with progressive neurological disease: regression of milestones of intellect, floppy, abnormal gait.
  (c) lymphoid interstitial pneumonitis.
  (d) recurrent protracted bacterial infections such as meningitis, pneumonia, internal organ abscesses, respiratory tract sepsis (discharge from ears or nose).
  (e) those with secondary cancers (rare) or other conditions such as hepatitis, kidney problems, or cardiomyopathy.

At the present time children are monitored for up to five years before they can be declared free from infection (and risk).

Immunisation

Thus far, the evidence is that routine childhood immunisation programmes are safe. BCG should not be given to symptomatic children, but generally this is not a problem since BCG is given just after birth when the child is not symptomatic. It is also recommended that attenuated polio vaccine is used rather than live vaccine as this is excreted in the feces and if an immunocompromised adult comes into contact with this (say during a nappy change), then there may be a risk of polio infection. It is useful to check the vaccination history of the parents. As our knowledge grows about the effects of HIV on children then this advice may be subject to change.

AZT and children

In September 1990, the US Federal Drug Administration (FDA) approved the use of AZT for children between three months to 12 years. Previously its use had only been recommended for children who were 13 years and over.

There have been a number of trials of AZT in children with AIDS. It has been linked with weight gain, reduction in liver and spleen size, and improved immune function. Parks and Abramowitz[54] reported that trials of AZT in children are finding increased growth rates and improved survival among children with AIDS so treated. AZT for children is available as a strawberry flavoured syrup.

Telling children, siblings and others

As children get older the question emerges, 'When should they be told about their HIV infection?' This is a difficult question and one where parents will make the decision based on their own beliefs, the treatments available, and the level of outside support for both them and their children. Parents need to be prepared for questions from the child about their illnesses and recurrent hospital visits. They may well have to cope with the child's anger – directed towards them, others, or turned in on the child him- or herself. It may be more constructive to tell the child as soon as possible so that they can assimilate the knowledge into their developing concept of who they are. But this is easier said than done and in practice many parents try to blank it out.

According to Mok,[48] school children who are HIV-positive should not be identified to schools unless they develop AIDS. If they do develop AIDS, then the teacher should be told in confidence in order to protect the child from possible infections from classmates. However, the parents of other children should not be informed. There may well be fears about discrimination from other children.

Caring for a terminally ill child can put parents and other family members under enormous strain. It is likely to have a detrimental impact on the stability of the parents' drug use. Resentment may emerge among any other children in the family because of all the attention that the child with AIDS receives. However, one beneficial outcome is the increased support that can be provided due to HIV, and IDU parents may be better able to care for their sick child than children they have had previously. Sue was able to look after her child, Mark, when he developed AIDS, and she nursed him at home. Her older son by a different father, Joe, lived with Sue's mother. She was using drugs heavily when she had him and saw him only occasionally. Joe resented this and would go round to Sue's house and cause arguments about why she could not 'do things like this for him? What was so special about Mark?' This is also true for children born when the parents are actually on drugs and those born when they are off drugs. The different quality of care can lead to resentment, 'Why wasn't I cared for like this?'.

Role reversal can take place among children of drug using parents. The children try to protect the parents and take care of them. When June, for example, started to get morning sickness due to her pregnancy, her 15-year-old son, Alan, started to refuse to go to school and stayed at home (previously he had been a regular attender). When confronted with this he admitted that he thought she was vomiting due to starting to use heroin again. June had not told him about the pregnancy. He had stayed home to keep an eye on her.

Foster care and adoption

Considering who will take care of your children after your death is an issue most people would not want to consider in too much detail. Drug users are no exception to this. The IDU's parents may not be a viable option if they are elderly. 'My mother's already looked after two of mine, she's getting too old to manage now, she certainly won't be able to take on another one.' Another reaction we have observed is, 'I know what my parents did to me and there's no way I'd want either of them looking after my kid'. When the parents are asymptomatic they seldom want to make definite plans even if they develop AIDS since this issue is often too painful for them to confront. The machinery for this process needs to be established before it is required. The difficulties need to be anticipated as far as possible. Where young children are put up for adoption, not knowing the child's antibody status can cause significant delays in placement.

The effect of HIV on children, and its implications for those involved in caring for them, are complex and wide ranging. It is not possible in the context of this book to consider them in any detail.

References

1. Chin, J., Sankaran, G. & Mann, J.M. (1989) Mother to infant transmission of HIV: an increasing global problem. In *Maternal and Childcare in Developing Countries,* (Eds. E. Kessel, A.K. Awan) Thun, Switzerland.
2. Mok, J. (1991) HIV infection and children. *British Medical Journal,* **302**, 921–2.
3. Boland, M. (1989) Ethical and legal concerns in developed countries. The implications of AIDS for mothers and children. Acts of the International Conference, Paris, 63–9.
4. Mann, J. (1989) Women, children and the global AIDS strategy. The implications of AIDS for mothers and children. Acts of the International Conference, Paris, 31–7.
5. Mulleady, G., White, D., Philips, K. & Cupitt C. (1990) Reducing sexual transmission of HIV for injecting drug users: the challenge for counselling. *Counselling Psychology Quarterly*. **3**, (4), 325–41.
6. Fraser, A.C. (1972) Drug addiction in pregnancy. *Proceedings of the Royal Society of Medicine,* **65**, 876.
7. Pelosi, A.M., Sana, J.C., Caterini, H. & Kaminetzky, H.A. (1974) Galactorrhea – amenorrhea syndrome associated with heroin addiction. *American Journal of Obstetrics and Gynaecology,* **118**, 966.
8. Cuskey, W.R. & Wathey, R.B. (1982) Female addiction: a longitudinal study. Lexington, Massachusetts: Lexington Books.
9. Apgar, V. (1966). The drug problem in pregnancy. *Clinical and Obstetric Gynaecology,* **9**, 623.
10. Ryder, R.W., Nsa, W., Behels, F., Vercauteren, G., Baendl, E., Lubaki, M., Baudeux, M., Quinn, T. & Piot, P. (1988) Perinatal transmission in two African hospitals: one year follow-up. IV International Conference on AIDS, Stockholm. (Abstract 4128.)
11. Levy, J., Puissant, F., Soumenkoff, G., Clumeck, N., Zissis-Sprecher, S., *et al.* (1988) Prospective study of the vertical transmission of HIV. IV international conference on AIDS. Stockholm. (Abstract 6582.)
12. Willoughby, A., Mendez, H. & Hittelman, J. (1988) Epidemiology of perinatal transmission of Human Immunodeficiency Virus. IV International Conference on AIDS. Stockholm. (Abstract 6588.)

13. Wilson, G.S., Desmond, M.D. & Wait, R.B. (1981) Follow up of methadone treated and untreated narcotic dependent women and their infants: health developmental and social implications. *The Journal of Paediatrics*, **98**, (5), 716–22.
14. Blatman, S. (1980) *Methadone effects on pregnancy and the newborn*. Dartmouth Medical School. (Unpublished.)
15. Finnegan, L.P. (1975) Narcotic dependency in pregnancy. *Journal of Psychoactive Drugs*, **7**, 299.
16. Williams, Ann (1985) When the client is pregnant: information for counsellors. *Journal of Substance Misuse Treatment*, **2**, 27–34.
17. Kreek, M.J. (1983) Clinical perinatal and developmental effects of methadone; critique. 15: Research on the treatment of narcotic addiction, state of the art. National Institute on Drug Abuse, Rockville, Maryland, 444–53.
18. Tylden, E. (1983) Care of the pregnant drug addict. *Mims magazine*, 1 June, 61–83.
19. Zuspan, F.P. (1976) Urinary amine alternations in drug addiction pregnancy. *American Journal of Obstetrics and Gynaecology*, **126**, (7), 955–64.
20. Blinick, G., Jerez, E. & Wallach, R.C. (1973) Methadone maintenance, pregnancy and progeny. *Journal of the American Medical Association*, **225**, 477.
21. Priestly, B.C. (1973) Drug addiction and the newborn. *Developmental Medicine and Child Neurology*, **15**, 200.
22. Connaughton, J.F., Reeser, D., Shut, J. & Finnegan, L.P. (1977) Perinatal addiction: outcome and management. *American Journal of Obstetrics and Gynaecology*, **129**, 679.
23. Chappel, J.N. (1972) Treatment of morphine type dependence. *Journal of the American Medical Association*, **221**, 1516.
24. Strauss, M.E., Ostrea, E.M. & Starr, R.H. (1976) Behavioural concomitants of perinatal addiction to narcotics. *Journal of Paediatrics*, **89**, (5), 842.
25. Finnegan, L.P., Connaughton, I.F. & Schut, F. (1975) Family center, a comprehensive programme for pregnant drug dependent women and their newborn. *Paediatric Research* (Baltimore), 9/4. No. 650.
26. Newman, R.C., Bashkow, S. & Calko, D. (1975) Results of 313 consecutive live births of infants delivered to patients in New York City methadone maintenance treatment programme. *American Journal of Obstetrics and Gynaecology*, **121**, (2), 233–37.
27. Blinick G., Wallach, R.C., Jerez, E. & Ackermann, B.E. (1976) Drug addiction in pregnancy and the neonate. *American Journal of Obstetrics in Gynaecology*, **125**, 135.
28. Finnegan, L.P. (1979) In utero opiate dependence and sudden infant death syndrome. *Clinical Perinatology*, **6**, 163.
29. Zelson, L., Lee, S.F. & Casalino, M. (1973) Neonatal narcotic addiction. Comparative effects of maternal intake of heroin and methadone. *New England Journal of Medicine*, **289**, 1216.
30. Glass, L. (1971) Absence of respiratory distress syndrome in premature infants of heroin addicted mothers. *Lancet*, **2**, 685.
31. Chasnoff, I.J., Burns, W.J. & Schnoll, S.H. (1985) Cocaine use in preg-

nancy. *New England Journal of Medicine*, **313**, (11), 666–9.

32. Bingol, N., Fuchs, M., Diaz, V., Stone, R.K. & Gromisch, D.S. (1987) Teratogenicity of cocaine in humans. *Journal of Paediatrics*, **110**, (1), 93–6.
33. Bashore, R.A., Ketchum J.S., Staisch, K.J., *et al.* (1981) Heroin addiction and pregnancy – Interdepartmental Clinical Conference. *Western Journal of Medicine*, **134**, 506–14.
34. MacCallum, L. (1988) Medical facts as they affect women. Women and AIDS Conference: Needs, Issues, Awareness. Edinburgh, 9–11.
35. Fried, P.A., Barnes, R.N., Drake, B.A. & E.R. (1985) Soft drug use after pregnancy compared to use before and during pregnancy. *American Journal of Obstetrics and Gynaecology*, **151**, 787–92.
36. Stauber, M., Schwerdt, M. & Tylde, E. (1983) Pregnancy, birth and puerperium in women suffering from heroin addiction. *Journal of Psychosomatic Obstetrics and Gynaecology*, 1–3/4, 128–38.
37. Ryder, R.W. & Hassig, S.E. (1988) The epidemiclogy of perinatal transmission of HIV. *AIDS*, **2**, (Suppl 1), 583–9.
38. Bledsoe, K., Poenia, O.L., Barnes, F., Delapenha, R., Saxinger, C. & Frederick W. (1990) The effect of pregnancy on progression of HIV infection. VI International Conference on AIDS, San Francisco.
39. Berrebi, A., Puel, J. Tricore, J., Herne, H. & Pontonnier, G. (1990) Influence of gestation on HIV infection. VI International Conference on AIDS, San Francisco.
40. Robertson, J.R., Skidmore, C.A., Roberts, J.J.K. & Elton, R.A. (1990) Progression to AIDS in IVDU co-factors and survival. VI International Conference on AIDS, San Francisco.
41. European Collaborative Study (1991) Children born to women with HIV-1 infection: natural history and risk of transmission. *Lancet*, **337**, 253–60.
42. Goedert, J.J., Duliège, A.M. & Amos, C.I. (1991) High risk of HIV-1 infection for first-born twins. *Lancet*, **338**, 1471–75.
43. Logan, S., Newell, M.L., Ades, T. & Peckham, C.S. (1988) Breast feeding and HIV infection. *Lancet*, **1**, 1346.
44. Howie, P.W., Forsyth, J.S., Ogston, S.A., Clark, A. & Florey, C.D. (1990) Protective effect of breastfeeding against infection. *British Medical Journal* **300**, 11–16.
45. Pokrovsky, V. & Keznepsova, I. (1990) Transmission of HIV infection from an infected infant to his mother by breast feeding. VI International Conference on AIDS, San Francisco. (Abstract Thc 831.)
46. Borkowsky, W., Krasinski, K., Paul, D., Lawrence, R., Chandwani, S., Moore, T. & Bebrenoth, D. (1988) Human immunodeficiency virus core protein antigenemia in children with HIV infection. IV International Conference on AIDS, Stockholm. (Abstract 7262.)
47. Rogers, M. (1988) Prospective study of urologic parameters for infants born to HIV seropositive women. IV International Conference on AIDS, Stockholm. (Abstract 7257.)
48. Mok, J. (1986) HIV seropositive babies – implications in planning for their future. In *The Implications of AIDS for Children in Care*. British Association for Adoption and Fostering, London.
49. Wieblen, B.J., Lee, F.K., Cooper, E.R., Sheldon, H.L., McIntosh, K.,

Harris, J.S., *et al.* (1990) Early diagnosis of HIV infection in infants by detection of IgA HIV antibodies. *Lancet*, **335**, 988–90.

50. Marshall, G.S., Barbour, S.D. & Plotkin, S.A. (1987) AIDS in a child with no antibody to HIV. *Lancet*, **1**, 446–7.
51. Laure, F., Courgnaud, V., Rouzioux, C., *et al.* (1988) Detection of HIV-1 DNA in infants by means of the polymerase chain reaction. *Lancet*, **ii**, 538–40.
52. Johnstone, F.D., Brettle, R.P., MacCallum R., Mok, J., Pentherer, F. & Burns, S. (1990) Women's knowledge of their HIV antibody state: its effect on their decision whether to continue the pregnancy. *British Medical Journal*, **300** (6th Jan.), 23–4.
53. Selwyn, P.A., Carter, R.J., Schoenbaum, E.E., Robertson, V.J., *et al.* (1989) Knowledge of HIV antibody status and decisions to continue to terminate pregnancy among intravenous drug users. *Journal of the American Medical Association*, **261**, 3567–72.
54. Parks, W.P. & Abramowitz (1989) Management of sero-positive mothers and children. The implications of AIDS for mothers and children. Proceedings of the International Conference, Paris, 213–18.

Chapter 9

Community Issues

Introduction

The transient nature of the drug-using population has implications for care when the IDU becomes ill. They may not have a network of people who can care for them or sustain them in the community. They will have to rely heavily on community support services.

Housing

Many clients are in local authority accommodation. Those on the waiting list (if they are lucky) will be in bed and breakfast accommodation. In the St Mary's study 32% of the sample were in bed and breakfast accommodation.[1] When asked to rate satisfaction with their current accommodation 44% were either not at all or only slightly satisfied.

In the London area, due to the shortage of council housing, clients may have to stay in bed and breakfast hotels for long periods of time (a period of at least one year was not unusual for clients attending St Mary's).

There will be a number of difficulties in delivering community nursing care to the client living in bed and breakfast, apart from the obvious practical ones. It may be difficult to provide discreet home nursing care in a crowded hotel, making confidentiality problematic. Frequently, the accommodation is small and cramped and the hotels crowded with families. The client does not always have an ensuite bathroom and toilet; if they are suffering from symptoms like diarrhoea then this is obviously unacceptable. Often cooking facilities are inadequate or there are no cooking facilities. This means that the client may not bother to eat or eats out and tends to eat cheap fast foods – not a good scenario if the client has a weight loss problem or a nutritional disorder. Whatever the food purchased, there is also the expense involved. For many of these reasons, IDUs who are admitted to hospital for in-patient care tend to occupy their beds longer than other patients if there is no suitable accommodation to discharge them to.

Squats or privately rented properties can be similarly unsuitable. Eileen, an HIV-positive drug user, and her one-year-old child, lived in a privately rented one-bedroomed flat. While watching a horror film on the TV one evening, her neighbour decided to drop in – through the ceiling! She said that she had seen some horror films in her day, but they were nothing compared to her neighbour's entrance.

Council housing is allocated on a points system, on the basis of an assessment of need. If the IDU's housing situation is threatening their stability or psychological well being, then they may be assessed as vulnerable; this will depend on local criteria operating. Being HIV-positive and asymptomatic may not gain the client any priority, but being symptomatic or having a diagnosis of AIDS generally does. Priority needs may be assessed on the following basis:

- pregnancy;
- having children;
- vulnerability as a result of old age, mental illness or disability;
- homelessness or threat of homelessness.

The worker should attempt to provide as much supportive written evidence as possible. Harassment, the threat of violence, and home conditions detrimental to health will also be taken into account. Housing agencies are very useful in arguing these issues in an appropriate manner. With the client's consent, the worker can write letters of support to the relevant housing departments, providing confirmation of the client's attendance at the agency, the nature of contact with the agency, HIV-diagnosis, current state of health, and any special needs they may have, the need for a ground floor flat, for example, disabled access, adequate heating, etc. Experienced housing advisors can be very useful, whether agency-based or located in local housing advisory centres.

Clients often get into difficulties through non-payment of bills. No one can be evicted without a court order. If this happens, they should stay put and try to get advice from solicitors, housing aid centres, organisations like Immunity (London-based), the Terrence Higgins Trust's legal advice line, or local HIV/AIDS advice agencies.

If the client is sharing council accommodation with a partner, it is best to have a joint tenancy. A legal or common law spouse has the right to carry on living in the property if the tenant leaves or dies (this also applies to any family member who has lived there for a year if there is no spouse). It is best to have the tenancy in joint names, particularly in same gender relationships. However, problems can arise if the relationship splits up as either tenant can surrender their rights. When a partner dies, councils sometimes have a policy of giving the survivor special rights. Housing advisors can be very helpful in assisting the client to make the appropriate decisions and helping with any problems that may arise.

There are now a number of housing agencies who deal specifically with letting properties to people affected by HIV. Accommodation is in demand from these agencies and getting someone a place can take time. There is a scarcity of accommodation for mothers with children as many of these flats are one-bedroomed.

Welfare eligibility

The person with AIDS will be eligible to apply for a range of benefits and community services. We are no longer entitled to welfare but, eligible (or not) to apply for benefits. Each case is then assessed. The IDU, for example, needs to be getting unemployment/sickness benefit before being eligible for assistance with rent/or community charges. These payments are discretionary and may not be 100% of the rent. The services available will vary depending on the area where the client lives. They may be provided by the local authority or council, hospital, charities, or community groups. Help can be obtained with the following:

- equipment and adaptations in the home, e.g. washing machines, mattresses, telephones;
- home care such as home helps, collecting prescriptions;
- meals and shopping, e.g. meals on wheels;
- transport such as taxicard scheme, mobility allowance.

Care in the community can put enormous burdens on the partner or family member; seeing a partner or family member becoming more debilitated; trying to cope with this, in some cases knowing they themselves are also HIV-positive; having a drug problem to deal with. The carer in the community is therefore a crucial resource. Clients and carers should be encouraged to make use of respite care facilities and any local community support. However, disability may not be a gradual process and may strike in a sudden, unpredictable way. This can make planning almost impossible, and the client will require urgent assessment and access to the necessary aids and benefits if this happens.

Specialist social workers and welfare rights workers can help with seeing that clients are getting all the benefits they are eligible for. It is as well to realise that this sort of help is often the client's primary concern. If you can assist them it will go a long way to engaging them. Some workers may feel that it is an inappropriate use of the worker's time and skills. More importantly, this may not be your area of expertise so that liaison and referral are essential. Even so, it can be an extremely frustrating and time-consuming experience for you and your client to try to sort out financial issues. Where non-payment of bills is concerned, they often leave the situation until it becomes a crisis and are threatened with services being cut off or eviction and only then do they seek outside assistance. This makes the situation even more difficult, but it is essential that the client is enabled to go some way to organising the solution themselves. Otherwise the situation will only be repeated. Again, clients can and do take advantage of the system wherever they can. Nigel, for example, used his mobility allowance to buy a bike. He also wanted a letter from his worker to take to the electricity board saying he was HIV-positive in the hope that this would get him out of paying his bill. Arrangements for instalment repayments can usually be made and some support organisations will help with bills. If money is going to change hands, especially, large sums, it is essential to ensure that it is spent on what it was intended for; safeguards must be built in such as making cheques for specified articles payable at specified suppliers, or requesting proof of purchase.

HIV-related disability

Many drug agencies are located in inappropriate, inaccessible places for disabled people. If the client becomes increasingly disabled as a result of HIV, then this issue will be of greater importance. It is not until you get a client with PCP struggling up a flight of stairs, or attempt to negotiate a wheelchair through your agency's narrow front door, that you realise this. If it is possible to make modifications to your unit for disabled access then do so.

The client may go through a grieving process as a result of decreased mobility and disablement. Disability can force them into situations they would otherwise be able to avoid. One client got mugged whilst trying to score some drugs, was knocked to the ground, and had both his drugs and money stolen. Due to the advanced stage of his illness he was unable to fight back. He was no longer able to score heroin and could not obtain an injectable prescription. Collection of medication for drug users from chemists needs to be sorted out when mobility is reduced. Some clinics operate an ID card scheme where, with the agreement of the pharmacist and clinic, a designated relative or friend collects the client's methadone for a set period of time. Obviously it is important that this relative or friend be reliable. Sometimes community nursing staff have done this or, if they have transport, have taken the client to collect their own drugs. The other alternative is to allow clients to collect their medication for extended periods of time in one go. Sometimes this works, but one client was ripped off on three separate occasions by friends who came round to see him and discovered where his methadone was hidden. This poses enormous problems since, generally, once a controlled drug has been dispensed, it will not be replaced. It is as well to keep the intervals as short as is convenient for the client and limited in terms of attracting others to the possibility of a sizeable amount of drugs.

Periods of imprisonment

Because of their involvement in a range of illegal activities (shoplifting, theft, etc.) many IDUs will spend time in prison. There is no drug treatment available in prisons for drug users nor are condoms or syringes and needles available under current policies. In the 1990 St Mary's study,[1] 70% of clients had been to prison; 83% had used drugs while they were there; 20% had shared works and 17% had had sex. Of the 17% who had sex in prison, only one was able to use a condom. This was a male prostitute who had condoms smuggled in for him by a member of the prison staff. There is much debate about HIV policies in prisons. Clearly, inmates practising high risk behaviours are at increased risk of HIV while in prison. Dolan *et al.*[2] found that syringe sharing in prison was at a higher rate than in the community. The IDU may be at higher risk of HIV in the prison setting.

Our group found some evidence that IDUs were able to change their usual route of administration of heroin from injecting to oral use (smoking). However, many workers have heard a great deal of convincing anecdotal evidence of prisons where one set of works is passed around a prison wing and when blunt is sharpened on a box of matches. One client described in detail how he had attempted to boil water to clean a set of works by breaking a razor, attaching each piece to a wire inserted in the socket of a plug and then putting these two 'live' blades into a glass of water to make it boil. An ingenious, but extremely dangerous expedient to be forced to take.

A further concern is the medical care that people with symptomatic HIV infection may require when in prison. For some of the more serious drug-related offences, clients may receive sentences that are likely to exceed their expected life spans. The overwhelming majority of prison medical facilities are insufficiently equipped or staffed to cope with caring for the terminally ill. Some prisons, however, like Saughton in Scotland, are attempting to do this – they have recently developed a 35-bedded unit for short-term offenders who are terminally ill. Some prisons will go to great lengths to ensure that the client gets the medical care they require: Eileen, for example, was receiving Interferon injections at the DDU in conjunction with her methadone collection in order to ensure that she had both on a regular basis. She was arrested and imprisoned for shoplifting. She was escorted to the DDU from the prison by taxi with two wardens, had her injection, and was taken back again. In other cases prisoners have not received their medical treatment, and suffer unnecessarily as a result, despite requests from professionals involved in their care.

As a result of viral infectivity regulations (VIR) in prisons, there are consequences for individual prisoners in making their HIV status known. These will usually involve segregation, and, in some cases, isolation from other prisoners. In one prison, before desegregation, two people had been identified as HIV-positive. After desegregation, on a single day in 1989, 26 inmates identified themselves as HIV-positive.[3] This change in policy came about as a result of decisions reached by the prison staff following HIV and AIDS training. Training and education of staff is essential in order to encourage enlightened policy changes. Being kept in isolation, served food on paper plates, and not allowed to exercise with other inmates, is totally unacceptable for people infected by HIV. It is something that many clients have had to endure.

Another problem is that of prescribing substitute drugs while someone is in prison. Although someone may be on a legitimate prescription for methadone, once imprisoned this may be stopped and the prisoner will be withdrawn from all drugs, often without any medication to lessen withdrawal symptoms.

Even if clients are not imprisoned or are held in custody, they may experience considerable trauma as a result of arrest. Bridget, for instance, an HIV-positive IDU, with her baby, was arrested for alleged shoplifting. They were taken into police custody and put in a cell. Her baby was then taken away from her and she was threatened that she would not get her back. She was frantic about this, and had to spend nine hours without her baby until the father was contacted (around midnight) and came to collect their one-year-old child. If IDUs have children and no partner or relatives able to look after them, their children may have to be taken into care. These periods of separation will be stressful for everyone concerned.

Prison visiting may not be a viable option for the drug worker due to staffing and time constraints. However, a number of organisations do have staff who will visit the client in prison and they can help with resettlement on release or support the client during their sentence. The probation officer is also an extremely useful person, having a role in both preventive and aftercare work, running support groups in both prison and community. There is usually little that can be done to prepare people for what might happen in prison although it is possible to talk with the client about the risks. Their previous experience (if any) can be a useful starting point and from here one may be able to discuss the possibility of transient sexual contacts and difficulties in practising both safer sex and safer drug use in this setting. Temporary use of safer routes of drug administration could be suggested, i.e. changing from injecting to oral use when in prison to provide some preparation for what might lie ahead of them. They also need to be warned about the dangers of overdosing on release from prison if they have been relatively drug-free during their time there.

Some HIV-positive clients have chosen to disclose their status to the courts in the hope that this will gain leniency for their sentencing. Having done this, one client was shocked to read in the local newspaper that her charges had been dropped because she had a 'terminal illness'. Newspaper reporters sometimes hang around the magistrates' courts in order to pick up newsworthy cases. Clients should be warned of this and solicitors need to be vigilant about confidentiality when they use this information.

References

1. Mulleady, G., White, D., Phillips, K. & Cupitt, C. (1990) Reducing sexual transmission of HIB for injecting drug users: the challenge for counselling. *Counselling Psychology Quarterly*, **3**, (4), 325–41.
2. Sexton, S. (1990) Prisons: another way. *AIDS Matters*, **2**, 5.
3. Dolan, K., Donoghue, M.C. & Stimson, C.V. (1990) Drug injecting and syringe sharing in custody and in the community: an exploratory survey of HIV risk behaviour. *The Howard Journal of Criminal Justice*, **29**, (3), 177–86.

Chapter 10

Diagnosis and Treatment of Opportunistic Infections

Introduction

The medical management of HIV disease covers the following four main areas:

(1) Antiviral – e.g. AZT to reduce HIV replication.
(2) Preventing opportunistic infections – to provide treatments that help prevent disease occurring – e.g. prophylactic pentamidine treatment.
(3) Recognition and treatment of opportunistic infections – regular follow-up and treatment when necessary.
(4) Management of tumours, should they occur, using radiotherapy or chemotherapy.

Prognostic tests

Prognostic laboratory tests are never carried out in isolation but usually combined with a physical examination; symptoms will also be monitored. The reason for this is that individuals can respond to these tests with a considerable degree of variation. Some people remain well for years despite getting discouraging test results.

It is helpful to have some knowledge of the diagnostic tests and treatments that exist for opportunistic infections because then you can enable the client to better understand what is happening to them in terms of their stage of HIV disease, and to prepare them for changes and to discuss possible treatment options.

It is sometimes necessary to explain to clients that tests of immune function can sometimes be quite misleading; they can be very discouraged after being told that their CD4 lymphocyte counts are low.

Tests vary in their predictive power; often they give more information about the person's immune functioning if they are carried out sequentially.

Prognostic tests are likely to be carried out after a positive antibody test in order to give a clearer indication of the person's immune functioning. The results of these tests may form the basis for treatment recommendations. Various blood tests will be carried out to examine the levels of blood cells and other constituents such as blood gases and cell subsets. In a healthy person, these will be between certain fixed levels – the degree to which the person with HIV deviates from this 'norm' will give an indication of the effect of HIV on their body and can also give signs about the types of infection they may have.

The tests which may be carried out include the following:

- CD4 lymphocyte counts;*
- p24 antigen;
- CD4/CD8 ratios;*
- CD8 cell count;
- serum interferon;
- serum IgA and IgE;
- core p24 antibody;
- B2 microglobulin levels;*
- neopterin levels;
- CMV IgG antibodies to explain some of the above further.

*denotes more commonly used markers.

CD4 lymphocytes (helper cell count)

This test counts the levels of CD4 white blood cells. The result gives an indication of the relative proportions of these cells which should be within certain fixed limits. The normal adult range is between 600–1700. In individuals where the level is greater than 600, this test will probably be repeated every six months. It will be done at shorter intervals, i.e. every 3–4 months if the level falls below 500, where treatment decisions may need to be made. AZT treatment may be suggested at levels below 500; *Pneumocystis carinii* pneumonia (PCP) proplylaxis may also be started at levels below 200. If the count falls below 200, the test may not be repeated once treatment has commenced, since this is one of the main functions of the test.

p24 antigen test

A major protein of HIV is known as p24. An increase in the level of p24 antigen is strongly related to progression to AIDS (a four-fold increase within three years). A positive result, therefore, in conjunction with other tests, will be used to decide if a course of treatment such as AZT is advisable. Antigen testing in conjunction with a positive HIV antibody result is becoming a routine procedure in some hospitals, as is testing for HIV-2. The levels of antibody produced to this protein decrease just before p24 antigen levels increase. A reduction in antibodies to this protein is also strongly indicative of disease progression.

Opportunistic infections and their treatment

The treatments and indeed the infections themselves will involve variable levels of intrusion into the individual's everyday life. Apart from the apparent cocktail of drugs the client sometimes has to take, the side effects of some drugs may mean that more medication needs to be taken to counteract adverse reactions. Frequently the types and dosages of drugs need to be juggled for each individual until maximum benefit and minimum discomfort can be achieved. This process can be unsettling and distressing for the client.

Pneumocystis carinii pneumonia (PCP)

As well as X-rays, investigations for PCP may include a procedure called bronchoscopy where a flexible tube with a camera is inserted into the bronchus and a small piece of tissue removed. This procedure can be uncomfortable and the patient may be offered a local anaesthetic of intravenous diazepam or other sedative to help them to relax during the procedure. (Diazepam also acts as a muscle-relaxant, aiding the passage of the bronchoscope.) This must be at an acceptable dosage for the IDU, otherwise they may not be able to tolerate the procedure. One client pulled the tube out because he maintained that he could feel it going down and it was hurting him. Midazolam may be given to block memory of the procedure. It is wise to tell the client that the staff carrying out this procedure may be wearing gowns, glasses and masks because if they are not expecting this, they can sometimes react badly to it.

Testing for blood gases gives indices of the relative levels of oxygen and other gases (e.g. carbon dioxide) in the blood. This requires an arterial blood sample and IDUs can get anxious about this because they are so familiar with the dangers and discomfort of hitting an artery when they inject drugs. Use of a local anaesthetic can be reassuring. A respiratory function test measures the vital capacity or breathing capacity of the lungs. It involves breathing in and out of a measuring device. A decrease in performance may give an early indication of lung problems.

Drug treatments for PCP include the use of Septrin, Trimethoprin, Dapsone or Pentamidine. Septrin may be given in intravenous or oral form. Pentamidine is used in some cases where an individual is allergic to the other drugs. It can be administered intramuscularly, a procedure which the patient may find painful. It may be also given prophylactically, or to prevent the development of PCP. This may involve home treatment or the client going to the hospital or clinic every couple of weeks and inhaling an aerosol of the drug through a mask for about an hour. This can be disruptive to the lifestyle of the client and he or she also needs to be organised enough not to miss appointments. It is unclear so far whether it is better to use general oral antibiotics or inhaled Pentamidine as a preventative measure. PCP can develop outside the lungs and this may be more likely if inhalers are used. With general oral antibiotics, infections like toxoplasmosis may also be controlled.

Candida

A gastroscopy may be necessary to diagnose candida infection in the upper end of the gut. Again, this involves the passage of a fibre-optic tube down the oesophagus. An injection of Valium may be administered beforehand to relax the patient. Treatment includes Ketoconazole tablets (these can cause a skin rash), Nystatin syrup; Fungilin lozenges or Fluconazole may also be used. The latter has fewer side effects than Ketoconazole. When thrush is recurrent Ketoconazole maintenance therapy is usually necessary. Drugs may be prescribed for gum diseases common among IDUs.

Bacterial infections

Bacterial infections such as salmonella and shigella will require rapid antibiotic treatment with, for example, ampicillin, taken either by injection or in tablet form.

Neurological symptoms

Neurological symptoms caused by the direct effect of HIV on brain tissue are treated by anti-viral drugs that cross the blood brain barrier. AZT (Zidovudine) is one of the few drugs shown to be able to do this. One outcome of improved treatment for people with AIDS is that in some cases life expectancy is increased. Some practitioners believe that symptoms like neurological problems and HIV-related dementia will be more common as a result. This will have important implications for care and management. The personality changes, emotional unpredictability and loss of functioning that can result can be extremely distressing both for the client and for their family and friends. There is the additional problem of diagnosing neurological problems when the client has used drugs.

Cancers and tumours

With Kaposi's sarcoma no treatment may be required (other than cosmetic camouflage) if it occurs on the skin surface. If it occurs elsewhere in the body then it may be treated by radiation or chemotherapy which carry side effects of nausea, hair loss, etc. A biopsy is first taken to confirm the type of tumour. Human papilloma virus (the wart virus) may be associated with cervical cell abnormalities in women, so routine smear tests and screening for STDs should be offered.

Abnormalities in cells of the cervix will be investigated by the smear test, in which the doctor removes a small sample of cells with a spatula. This involves pelvic examination which some women can find distressing. It depends very much on the staff's sensitivity to this and their ability to reassure the client. If there is evidence of severe abnormalities then a cone biopsy will be carried out. A small piece of tissue is removed by a laser incorporated in a magnifying instrument called a colposcope. This is a fairly painless procedure and there are usually no symptoms apart from a slight discharge of blood. If there is evidence of malignancy then surgery may be required. Usually this involves hysterectomy (removal of the womb). Subsequent chemotherapy may be necessary.

Toxoplasmosis

Toxoplasmosis is a condition of enlarged glands, fever, and brain abscesses; it is caused by a protozoan parasite. This condition is diagnosed by brain scan. A brain or CT scan is a specialised form of X-ray. It is painless and sometimes a dye is injected beforehand to highlight the areas of soft tissue that are affected.

Treatment involves pyrimethamine by injection or in tablet form. The client may be put on a maintenance dose of this. It can cause anaemia in some patients.

Cryptococcal meningitis

This condition, inflammation of the meninges of the brain, can be diagnosed by lumbar puncture. A needle is inserted into the spinal canal in the lumbar region. The pressure of the fluid is measured and a sample of the spinal fluid collected. This procedure is quick but can be uncomfortable. The patient has to lie flat for about 24 hours afterwards to avoid developing a headache. Treatment of infection is by a course of intravenous amphotericin. This drug may have adverse effects on the kidneys.

Cytomegalovirus (CMV)

Among other things this virus can cause blindness. It is treated with DHMG (ganclyclovir). Again, after treating the acute infection, this drug may be given on a maintenance basis and involves injections three times a week. Occasionally an alternative anti-viral agent, Foscarnet, is used. Both drugs can cause anaemia.

Herpes

These are painful skin lesions which, depending on the type of virus involved, can occur around the mouth, genitals, anus or in the gullet.

The anti-viral drug acyclovir is used to treat and prevent the recurrence of herpes.

Thrombocytopenic purpura

This is a disorder in which there are too few platelets (blood clotting agents) and haemorrages arise from all mucosal surfaces. This condition is sometimes treated by removal of the spleen or with steroids. Intravenous gammaglobulin (an immune system stimulant) can lead to a temporary increase in the level of blood platelets.

Tuberculosis

Although the organism *Mycobacterium tuberculosis* can cause disease in every organ in the body, the most common site affected is the lungs. A person must have active, untreated TB in his or her lungs in order to infect others. It is for this reason that in the early stages of in-patient treatment for this disease, health care staff will probably wear masks since the patient is potentially infectious to others.

Infection with TB is lifelong but most people with intact immune systems can contain the infection and never develop the disease. The symptoms of TB can be easily confused with non-specific HIV-related symptoms (fever, malaise, weight loss). HIV-infected patients with TB sometimes have normal X-rays. Diagnosis depends on finding the organism in body secretions. TB can also be detected with a skin test. Treatment involves a combination of 3 or 4 drugs taken over 3 or 4 months.

In the United States in some settings that have daily contact with IDUs; in residential units and maintenance clinics, for example, daily antituberculosis chemotherapy has been given, sometimes in combination with methadone. However, these drugs can be toxic to the liver (e.g. Ioniazid) and in view of the high levels of liver problems among IDUs, close monitoring is required.

Other pneumonias

Pneumococcal or other bacterial infections have been found to be important early indicators of the subsequent HIV infection among IDUs.[1,2] Bacterial pneumonia, especially if it is recurrent, may be an indicator of HIV infection in the IDU.

One of the most common of the pneumonias is caused by *Streptococcus pneumoniae* (pneumococcus). Typically, the person becomes ill within one or two days, with high fever, marked shivering, and a cough producing yellow or green sputum. Chest pain associated with coughing or breathing and shortness of breath may also be present. This condition responds well to appropriate antibiotics such as penicillin or erythromycin. Several studies have indicated a positive response to pneumococcal vaccine among HIV-positive people.[3]

Hepatitis B

This infection was common among drug users prior to HIV. In some studies over 50% of IDUs showed evidence of hepatitis B exposure.[4,5] Unlike TB, there is no evidence that the course of hepatitis infection is altered by HIV, but it has been noted that replication of the virus which causes it, Hepatitis B virus (HBV), may be elevated and more persistent in HIV-positive IDUs and homosexual men.[6,7,8] Enhanced replication of Hepatitis Delta Virus (HDV) has also been seen in some individuals.[9] It makes sense for both IDUs and workers to have hepatitis B vaccinations to reduce transmission of HBV and HDV. Hepatitis can be tested for by a saliva test although a blood test is more reliable. If the IDU develops endocarditis (inflammation of the lining of the heart) it may also be more severe in those who are HIV-positive.[10]

Available treatments for HIV and AIDS

Anti-virals

Many drugs against HIV have come and gone. Often, claims for their therapeutic benefits have been made prematurely or inaccurately reported. There is considerable debate about whether test drugs should be released for clinical use sooner because of the possibility of their therapeutic benefits. There has been some relaxation of the rigorous and lengthy trial process that new drugs have to undergo as a result of successful campaigning by people with HIV and AIDS. The anti-viral drug that has received most attention is AZT. Work is also underway to test various combinations of these drugs: recent success using AZT and acyclovir is one example.

Producing the ideal anti-viral agent is a tall order. In order to be effective it requires the following:

- protects uninfected cells;
- reduces viral production from infected cells;
- is specific;
- is orally absorbed;
- crosses the blood-brain barrier;
- has no (or few) side effects.[1]

Anti-virals which have been or are still under investigation include Flourothymidine, Ampligion, AL721, Fucidin, Suramin, Foscarnet, Ribavirin, HPA23, DDC, Compound Q and Inosine pranobex.

AZT (Azidothymidine–Zidovudine–Retrovir

This drug was originally an anti-cancer drug, developed in the 1960s, but not used due to its toxicity. It works by inhibiting the action of the enzyme reverse transcriptase. This enzyme enables the RNA of HIV to be transformed into the DNA of the host cell.

In 1985 came the first suggestions that it might benefit the immune and nervous systems of people with AIDS. AZT was found to delay disease progression and allow a better quality of life – and prolonged survival – in people with AIDS. There were fewer opportunistic infections and weight gains; in addition, there was an abatement of neurological symptoms and patients reported greater energy levels. The problems with the drug were the side effects it caused in some patients – bone marrow suppression after 6 to 8 months, anaemia, neutropenia, muscle wasting and nausea. Approximately 50% suffer side effects, but these are less severe with HIV-asymptomatic patients. The cost of the drug is prohibitive. Obviously this factor restricts its availability. In addition, 20 to 30% of people who take it for two years or more develop resistance to it. Disease progression does continue despite AZT treatment, although the reasons for this are not yet clear.

AZT was licensed in the UK by the Department of Health in September 1990 for asymptomatic patients who are at high risk of developing infections, that is, those who have low T-cell (or CD4) counts persistently less than 200, or between 500–200 and falling rapidly.

The early use of AZT is controversial as some researchers feel that not enough is yet known about its long-term side effects and especially about AZT resistance. Lower doses are recommended but dosage guidelines are not universally agreed and there is uncertainty about the timing of treatment for best results. It is therefore unclear whether patients who are destined to remain well for many years would benefit from early treatment or treatment deferred until they eventually become symptomatic. The risks of early treatment include development of drug resistance by the virus and late development of toxicity to AZT. It is therefore controversial whether AZT should be offered to all asymptomatic patients.[11] Some of the benefits of AZT are temporary. Its long-term toxicity is not yet established. There are also major resource implications if early AZT treatment becomes the norm.

Many trials of this drug are in progress, and the UK and France trial of AZT in early infection continues. In the USA, at least 12 trials are testing a variety of combinations of other drugs with AZT. Much work is going on to establish what the optimal dosage is, especially in combination with other drugs like alpha interferon, dideoxycytidine (DDC) and dideoxyinosine (DDI). It is likely that AZT will eventually be used in combination with other drugs in order to enhance its effectiveness and reduce the toxicity (by enabling a lower dosage to be prescribed and earlier administration). Being in a drug trial can result in anxieties for the client as they may not know whether they are receiving the placebo or the drug. They may also have to undergo extensive monitoring of their physical condition. We found that many clients were unwilling to participate in a trial where they would not be guaranteed to receive AZT. This uncertainty is felt to be unacceptable, especially for individuals whose knowledge about drugs is often extensive and who usually know what they are taking (even if they are less aware of its purity). Most drug trials now have an option clause where, if the client is deteriorating and is found to be in the placebo condition, they will be given the option to cease treatment or go into the drug trial group. In some cases they can choose to go straight into the drug trial group, and in this case this can involve a comparison between different dosage levels or drug combinations.

It has been suggested that the effects of AZT may be altered by oral opiate administration with elevated plasma levels and reduced clearance of AZT. This was observed in a group of IDUs in Edinburgh who were taking methadone and/or DF118 along with AZT.[12] This finding is undergoing further investigation as it may have implications for higher AZT dosage levels for opiate-using clients.

There is also the problem of the image of AZT. It has become closely associated with AIDS, and as a result some clients are unwilling to take it, especially when they are asymptomatic, because it is a constant reminder of HIV. When clients do start taking it, it can have an enormous psychological impact. Possibly as a result of this they are sometimes inconsistent in taking the drug. Occasionally this feeling is manifested as a particular concern with the toxic side effects of AZT. Some medical staff have found this hard to understand considering the street drugs that IDUs may routinely take.

Women have until recently had very little involvement in drug trials. If drug-using women are to be included then some of these lifestyle issues need to be taken into consideration, including the fact that they are advised to avoid pregnancy once they are in the trial due to the possible toxicity to the fetus.

In the US AZT is now available for children (previously only for those over 13 years, now from 3 months–12 years). It is administered as a strawberry flavoured syrup.

DDI (Dideoxyinosine) is now being made available to some people with HIV-related diseases who are intolerant of AZT, and to those who are deteriorating on AZT. Its toxic side effects include peripheral neuropathy (numbness, burning sensation or pain in the feet) and inflammation of the pancreas (an organ whose enzymes metabolise fats, carbohydrates and sugars). DDI interferes with HIV's ability to encode its DNA into the genetic blueprint of the host cell. It is cheaper than AZT. Neurological and pancreatic damage is known to occur so far in about 1% of patients. This is fewer than the equivalent number who experience side effects with AZT, but the side effects of DDI are more serious. This makes it more likely that DDI will only be given to clients who for one reason or another cannot continue to take AZT. The alpha trial is the DDI drug trial for people who cannot tolerate AZT. The delta trial is a drug trial of combined AZT and either DDI or another drug, DDC. At the moment, DDI is only available to those on these drug trials or on compassionate release. It is not yet licensed in the UK.

Immune system stimulants (immunomodulators)

These are drugs which are used to improve or enhance the function of the immune system. They include drugs such as Interferon, Interleukin 2, and Imuthiol. Most immune-enhancing treatments in AIDS have focused on T4 cells – making them function properly, increasing their numbers, or protecting them from HIV infection. Many are in the process of being tested, often in combination with anti-viral medications.

Vaccines

There are significant doubts about whether a vaccine can ever be 100% effective against HIV because a person with HIV develops multiple variants of the virus. In addition, after introduction into the blood, the virus enters the T4 cells rapidly where it is resistant to most vaccines. However, significant steps have been made in vaccine development, so there is now more hope for this process.

The V3 loop is a small piece of the outer protein coat of HIV. Antibodies in the V3 loop appear to de-activate the virus. Although most researchers are agreed about this, the difficulty is that the sequences in the loop vary from one variant of HIV to another, so the antibodies might only protect against one strain of the virus. Work has begun to develop a cocktail vaccine using portions from four different types of HIV. Ultimately, it is thought that this could provide protection against up to 80–85% of known strains of the virus.

Vax Syn HIV aims to stimulate the killer cells of the immune system rather than stimulate antibodies. Attempts to inoculate monkeys with whole particles of Simian Immune Deficiency Virus found no trace of SIV six months later and none had the AIDS-like disease SIV normally causes. There are questions about whether the vaccine would give protection against other strains of HIV.

Although an effective vaccine is still a very long way off, there is now greater optimism about its development than there was five years ago.

Drug interactions

Certain medications in combination with each other can interact to negate the effect that, used singly, they were intended to produce.

The drug rifampicin, used for TB treatment, dramatically increases the excretion of methadone and reduces plasma methadone levels because of increased liver activity. The IDU may experience withdrawal within a few days of starting treatment. The daily dose of methadone therefore has to be increased to the order of 10 mg every 1 to 2 days (sometimes up to a level 50% higher than the original dose).[13] Sometimes methadone is divided into a twice-daily dose which helps to reduce symptoms that would otherwise occur at the end of a single daily dose.

Phenytoin is sometimes used to prevent seizures in people with AIDS who have central nervous system infection or other brain lesions, and has been shown to increase methadone metabolism through increased liver activity. Increases in methadone dosage do not, however, need to be as great as with Rifampicin.[14]

Self medication

There are occasions when clients may self-medicate either in combination with formal treatment or because they do not (for a variety of reasons) receive formal or regular medical care. Very often this involves treating their own abscesses (caused as a result of their injecting drug use), using, for example, Hirudoid cream which is manufactured for relieving the pain of haemorrhoids and varicose veins. It can help to relieve pain and encourage healing in veins that have become inflamed due to repeated injections. Clients also sometimes use topical antibiotic creams to treat their own abscesses. Obviously this can expose them to more serious infections as a result of unsterile technique. At the very least, not having abscesses properly cleaned and dressed, can lead to the development of deep pitted scar tissue on the body and to slow healing. Where medical and nursing care is available to drug users, abscesses are one of the most commonly treated physical problems. Clients may self medicate with antibiotics and other medications. It is not unknown for AZT to be sold to HIV-positive clients who are not receiving medical care or to IDUs just following an episode of needle sharing. If the client does present for health care and is about to embark on a course of treatment, it is important to find out what forms of self-treatment they have used and whether they do occasionally buy other medications as this may have important implications for drug interactions and toxicity.

In-patient care

Prior to HIV, many of the less serious physical problems experienced by IDUs – such as abscesses – resulted in their being best characterised as 'walking wounded'. Often they would treat themselves for the medical complications of their drug use. Admissions to hospital were usually for more serious conditions and often took place in situations of emergency – via the Accident and Emergency department, for example – for sub-bacterial endocarditis or serious overdose. As a result of this, many in-patient care staff have little or no regular experience of working with IDUs. With HIV, many more IDUs are going to require in-patient care.

Indirectly, the better access to health care now afforded to many IDUs is also likely to increase this need. In-patient care staff are going to see many more drug users and will need the co-operation and support of experienced drug workers (who should also benefit from a greater understanding of in-patient care priorities and service constraints). For example, the low socio-economic conditions of many IDUs is likely to have a direct impact upon the duration of in-patient stays. Delays in discharge may be brought about by poor access to adequate housing as well as interim and respite care.

Pain control

The following drugs are commonly used for pain control in hospitals: morphine, diamorphine, DF118, paracetamol and Temegesic. A variety of other medications may be used either singularly or in combination. A recent report by the Royal College of Surgeons stated that 'the treatment of pain after surgery in British hospitals has been inadequate and has not advanced significantly for many years'. Tolerance of pain is individual and varies enormously from person to person. IDUs are often very concerned that the level of pain killing drugs they will receive will be inadequate to meet their needs. If the levels of analgesia are not perceived to be high enough, or they feel they are withdrawing from the drug, then this can be a major contributory factor to the IDU 'topping up' with other drugs or taking their own discharge and leaving the hospital before treatment is completed. Generally, they will have an increased tolerance to pain killing drugs and will therefore require them at higher levels than are routinely administered. The client is much more likely to give a grossly inflated estimate of what he or she requires if they feel their needs are not going to be listened to (there may be a tendency to do this anyway).

Due to their awareness of the patient's drug use, staff are often much more vigilant about monitoring the levels of analgesia given to the IDU who can sometimes end up getting less medication than non-users. It can be enormously reassuring for the client to have some control over the levels of pain relieving medication they will receive. The morphine pump – used in some hospitals to control post-operative or terminal stage pain – is a good example of this. Every half hour or so the patient presses a button at their side and a small dose of morphine is automatically pumped into the bloodstream. A cutout switch prevents the button being pressed too soon after the previous dose. Morphine and diamorphine may also be given via tablet or injection.

Pain control is less likely to be an issue in the terminal stages of illness where liberal access to morphine-like drugs is allowed.

Hospice care staff are well aware of pain control management and are more used to the client having an active role in the negotiation of appropriate medication. Where this is less clear cut is where analgesia is required for post-operative pain or, in the earlier stages of illness, for symptom control. The dilemma occurs between not wanting to contribute to the IDUs drug problem and ensuring that they are comfortable. You do not really want the client to leave the hospital with a worse drug problem than when he or she came in. If the client is drug-free on admission, then the situation is even more delicate. Frequently the one thing the client has been in control of before going into hospital is the drugs they take. Even if they are on a prescription for drugs they may still choose to 'top up' when they are an out-patient. A common fear is that when they are admitted they have no control over this and have to rely on staff to be sympathetic to their needs.

It is helpful from the outset to allow the client some level of choice, but to recognise there are limits to this. The IDU is often very well informed; they are likely to know as much, if not more than staff, about the drugs that may be provided in hospital. Either ward staff or the drug worker should elicit information about what they think they need, compare it with their drug history, that is, duration of drug use, type used, quantities, compare it to what you would give a non-drug user, decide an approximate dosage, and gradually increase until they seem comfortable. But always tell them what you are going to do, the limits within which you will compromise, and bear in mind that they may well test the limits you have set so that you need to be clear why they are in place. Occasionally these limits are of the 'there's no reason for it, it's just our policy' variety. If they are, and it is a policy decided by staff consensus, then it is likely to be easier to defend. Obviously, contracting on the ward involves more than drug issues.

Although some loss of control for the client is inevitable, it is possible to enhance the areas where a negotiated compromise between staff and the client can be reached. It is here that liaison with a drug worker can be very helpful to staff unfamiliar with working with drug users. We may have a certain stereotype of the 'good patient' – co-operative, polite and grateful. To quote one ward sister, 'The staff are stretched to the limit as it is, one difficult client and we run into all sorts of problems.' Drug users (and indeed many other people) may not fit the 'good patient' bill, and as their behaviour is contrary to much of the previous experience in caring for people with AIDS, then they can sometimes end up on the receiving end of unworkable or punitive control measures.

Some degree of control is essential, but, basically, if the system is open to manipulation then don't blame the drug user for finding the loopholes. If limits are to be set about what is and is not acceptable behaviour, then the consequences of this must be workable and require the backing of management and of the medical staff. Contracting usually works better on paper than in practice and can be very difficult for ward staff to implement. There is no point in setting boundaries that are not adhered to. Inflexible ward policies tend to be labour intensive, an unacceptable situation for already over-burdened ward staff.

It is by no means always the case, but sometimes drug users can present management problems on the ward. Some of the issues that can emerge are as follows:

(1) Patients leaving the ward with Hickman catheters *in situ*. These are tubes which allow direct access to the right atrium of the heart. They are widely used with people with AIDS who require long-term intravenous infusions, antibiotics, chemotherapy, blood transfusions, total parenteral nutrition, and frequent blood sampling. The disadvantage of this for the IDU is that they could misuse the Hickman catheter by injecting unsterile drugs into it, thereby exposing themselves to serious infection risks. This would be especially appealing to someone whose veins were in very poor condition and who had trouble getting venous access. Health care staff may justifiably be anxious about using this procedure because of the risks. They are certainly less likely to use it for out-patient care. The disadvantage from the client's point of view is that frequent blood sampling may be a painful procedure for them because their veins are in poor condition.
(2) IDUs who are mobile may leave the ward for reasons other than visiting the league of friend's shop – for example, for dealing, scoring drugs, etc.
(3) Illicit drug use that the staff are unaware of may interfere with test results and lead to difficulties in interpretation of symptoms. There is also the risk of drug interactions which may be damaging to the IDU.
(4) The IDU is usually a heavy smoker and they will be unable to smoke on the ward.
(5) They may be unco-operative with treatment regimes: David, for example, had TB and was very unreliable in taking his medication. He insisted on taking it in his own time and not at the drug round. Eventually he stopped taking his medication outright because he was 'sick of being pushed around'. It was very difficult for staff to

see a patient deteriorate when this was not necessarily an inevitable consequence of his condition.

(6) The IDU can be demanding of staff time, but they can also respond positively to any signs of interest in their situation.

(7) They can sometimes disturb the other patients, cadging cigarettes and sometimes offering to relieve them of their sedative or pain killing drugs.

It can be very difficult for the IDU to be hospitalised; there is the loneliness and isolation – few of their friends may have telephones for them to be contacted by the patient. They may be stigmatised as a drug user – they are sometimes put in side wards or in cubicles away from the other patients on the ward. The fact that many of them sleep during the day and stay awake at night can increase this sense of isolation.

There are no clear cut answers to some of the management problems that will arise. In some cases it is a 'no win' situation and ward staff may be forced to turn a blind eye; indeed this may be the only option if the treatment regime requires in-patient care. A clear set of guidelines about working with drug users is required, especially if agency staff are employed. 'Shared care' is one solution. In-patient management problems can be exacerbated by staff who know little about drug users or drugs and where no drug workers are available. Training should be offered to staff unfamiliar with working with drug users – this will necessitate time off from the wards and needs accommodation from management.

Patients cannot be watched every minute of the day and night. Speaking to one ward sister about a drug-using patient elicited the following: 'he gets very bored; we can't stop his visitors. We've explained to him the need to avoid using drugs on top of his medication, but I guessed he was using occasionally'. The situation is often one of compromise: 'I explained that we didn't want him to withdraw from drugs and that we would do our best to ensure that he was comfortable. I also explained that topping up with non-prescribed drugs would interfere with making an accurate diagnosis.' Occasionally the client will tell you what they have used on top, particularly if they know you will be understanding about this. If you find the IDU taking illicit drugs try to clarify the reasons for this – is it insufficient medication? inappropriate medication? an unsuitable regime? One client, for example, took his methadone in two separate doses and liked to have some before going to sleep but the nursing staff were concerned about this as they usually dispensed the methadone in one daily dosage.

Tina was accused of getting drugs from her boyfriend because she slept most of the day. 'She doesn't understand I usually sleep most of the day and don't get up until the evening. I told her if she didn't believe me she could test my urine.' The drug Tina used was cocaine. This is unlikely to induce sleep in the user. She was also treated for scabies when in fact she was suffering from cocaine overdose and was scratching at her skin because she was convinced she was infected with 'crawly things'. This is a case that highlights the benefits of closer drug worker–ward liaison. For cocaine and amphetamine users, anxiolytic or sedative drugs can go some way to alleviating the withdrawal symptoms. Longer term pharmacologic interventions have included tricyclic antidepressants and other dopaminergic agents.[15,16]

At the very least, in-patient nursing and medical staff should be equipped to assess the nature and extent of illicit drug use. If the client goes into heroin withdrawal the symptoms will complicate the treatment because of their overlap with HIV-related conditions: diarrhoea, cramps, sweating and agitation. Further to this, the client is unlikely to hang around to suffer these symptoms and is therefore unlikely to comply with any treatment regimes which are necessary. There must also be clear communication between doctor and nursing staff. Doctors should not change substitute prescribing regimes without consulting with the nursing staff as well.

It can take a while for clients to get to know the medical and nursing staff. It is not unusual, due to rotation of medical staff, for the client to see a number of different staff over the course of the treatment. It can be distressing for the IDU who has got to know and trust their doctor and then has to get used to seeing someone new. This may lead to their becoming more passive and not asking for feedback about their treatment: such feedback and the results of their tests are both important.

If the client is already involved with a drug agency they may be concerned about liaison between the ward and the DDU and may be reluctant to admit to using on top of their prescription. If possible, the client may need to be reassured that divulging illicit use will not result in punitive measures and that any possible increase in medication required will be taken into account by the drug agency on discharge. This compromise may require the prescribing agency to start at a higher dosage and then gradually reduce to a level which is acceptable to their prescribing policies. The drug agency may not be willing to prescribe benzodiazepines, often given as night sedation on the ward, and the IDU may need to be made aware of this and the compromise arrangement reached by which a short-term reducing prescription is supervised by the drug agency following discharge. Flexibility in the prescribing policy can keep liaison problems to a minimum, but ward staff need to be aware that the client may still not wish the drug agency to know what they are really taking. DDUs should be prepared to take on new clients once they are discharged from the ward. If there is no DDU then liaison should start on admission either with the client's GP or with the local drug agency. For this reason, discharge of the patient should not take place on a Friday evening when it will not be possible to organise a script.

Many drug users find the ward a safe and comfortable place to be and can be reluctant to leave. Many of them may have no suitable accommodation to go to on discharge, something which can extend the length of their stay. It is necessary to involve the hospital social worker or welfare rights workers early on to assist with any accommodation problems the client might have.

Alternative and complementary therapies

Alternative, complementary, or holistic treatments encompass several different therapies.[17] These attempt to consider the person as a whole (mind, body and spirit) rather than in terms of the specific illness or illnesses, something which has tended to be the main Western medical tradition. The use of these therapies in the treatment of people with HIV and AIDS has grown considerably. Not all medical authorities are agreed on the value (if any) of these treatment approaches. While most appear to do no harm, it has been argued that their value lies mainly in suggestion or in promoting a generally more healthy attitude to life and an enhanced sense of personal control. More tangible evidence of their efficacy is needed, and until such time as it is, it is wise to exercise caution about the treatment methods chosen. Some methods have been much more extensively researched than others – autogenics, for example, yoga, acupuncture, etc. While others are plainly 'way out'. The client needs to distinguish between these.

Holistic treatment can encompass several different treatment modalities, including the following:

- conventional use of Western medicine including drugs, surgery or radiotherapy;
- the use of complementary methods such as homoeopathy, acupuncture, acupressure, herbal remedies, hypnotherapy, spiritual healing, naturopathy, reflexology, shiatsu;

- practising self-help skills such as breathing and relaxation techniques, meditation, visualisation, yoga, aromatherapy, autogenic training, physical exercise and diet.

Many IDUs express an interest in alternative medicine. Quite a number have expressed the desire to try hypnotherapy, frequently expressing their hope that they could be hypnotised to stop wanting to take drugs. The hope that we can bypass our own motivation to stop particular behaviours is not uncommon. Unfortunately, nothing is ever that simple.

Some clients who have become involved in alternative medicine have found it helpful. This kind of medicine may require considerable commitment on the part of the IDU whose involvement often takes the form of 'dabbling' with a particular method; regular practice is less commonly seen. Although interest may be sporadic, many clients are keen to try out these techniques. It is sometimes necessary to emphasise the complementary nature of these therapies: that they are an adjunct and not to be used to the exclusion of more conventional modes of treatment. This is important because sometimes an obsessive commitment to a particular therapy can lead the client to stop taking their conventional medications. Occasionally a client adopts one particular therapy and if they continue to get sick they may blame themselves, feeling that they have not 'done it properly'. Many drug workers have developed interests in this area and can offer some of the therapies 'on site': these include acupuncture, aromatherapy and shiatsu. Indeed, before HIV, many of the techniques were used with some success to alleviate the symptoms of drug withdrawal. Many training courses are available for workers who wish to find our more about these holistic medicines, but training as well as treatment may prove expensive – the essential oils used in aromatherapy, for example, can be costly.

At a more basic level, many workers become familiar with relaxation techniques. There are a wide variety of these – deep progressive relaxation, controlled breathing, imagery-based techniques, autogenic training, biofeedback. If the client shows a sufficient level of interest and commitment, then it can be useful to provide training in these techniques. They can be particularly useful in helping the client who is coming off drugs to cope with the increase in anxiety symptoms which inevitably seems to follow.

The benefits of different methods will vary from person to person and the client may need to shop around until they find one that suits them. If the client takes an interest in alternative therapies, one of the benefits can be an increased awareness of their body and the need to care for it. If alternative methods enhance the client's sense of control then so much the better.

Many practitioners offer a sliding financial scale for those in genuine financial hardship and in some settings these treatments are offered free to people with HIV and AIDS. Some alternative therapists work closely with more traditional health care services; a number of hospitals also have links with holistic therapists. It is important to establish that the practitioner is fully trained and what their credentials are (see resource list for further details).

Alternative therapies are systematically evaluated in terms of type of benefit derived, physical improvement, psychological improvement, or cure. This is an unfortunate feature of alternative therapy. There is also the fact that many of these treatments come and go like fashions. At the present time, the most pressing need for the IDU is adequate access to primary health care – there is still a long way to go before this basic requirement is fulfilled.

References

1. Selwyn, P.A., Feingold, A.R., Hartel, D., *et al.* (1988) Increased risk of bacterial pneumonia in HIV infected intravenous drug users without AIDS. *AIDS* **2**, 267–72.
2. Dobkin, J., Mandell, W. & Sethi, N. (1989) Bacteremic pneumococcal disease as the first manifestation of HIV infection in adults. V International Conferences on AIDS. Montreal (abstract MBP 71).
3. Huang, K.L., Rube, F.L., Rinaldo, C.R., *et al.* (1987) Antibody responses after influenza and pneumococcal immunisation in HIV infection homosexual men. *Journal of the American Medical Association*, **257**, 2047–50.
4. Stimmel, D., Vernace, S. & Schaffner, F. (1975) Hepatitis B surface antigen and antibody. A prospective study in asymptomatic drug abusers. *Journal of the American Medical Association*, **243**, 1135–8.
5. Kreek, M.J., Dodes, L., Kane, S., *et al.* (1972) Long-term methadone maintenance therapy: effects on liver function. *Annals of Internal Medicine*, **77**, 598–602.
6. Sinicco, A., Valle, M., Santoro, A., *et al.* (1989) Correlation between HIV and HBV infection. V International Conference on AIDS, Montreal (Abstract MBP 219).
7. Rossol, S., Voth, R., Meyer sum Biischenfelde, K.H. & Hess, G. (1989) Modulation of viral hepatitis in HIV-1 infection. V International Conference on AIDS, Montreal (Abstract MBP 220).
8. Bodworth, N. & Donovan, B. (1989) The effect of HIV on chronic hepatitis B: a study of 150 homosexual men. V International Conference on AIDS, Montreal (Abstract MBP 222).

9. Lake-Baharr, G., Bhat, K. & Goundaragjan, S. (1989) HIV infection and delta hepatitis in intravenous drug addicts. V International Conference on AIDS, Montreal (Abstract MBP 218).
10. Selwyn, P.A. (1989) Issues in the clinical management of intravenous drug users with HIV infection. *AIDS*, **3**, (Suppl 1): S201–S208.
11. Volberding, P.A., Lagakos, S.W., Koch, M.A., *et al.* (1990) AIDS Clinical Trials Group of the National Institute of Allergy and Infectious Diseases. Zidovudine in asymptomatic human immunodeficiency virus infection. *New England Journal of Medicine*, **322** (14), 941–9.
12. Brettle, R.P., Jones, G.A., Bingham, J., *et al.* (1989) Pharmacokinetics of zidovudine in injecting drug use related HIV infection. V International Conference on AIDS, Montreal (Abstract WB 03).
13. Selwyn, P.A. (1989) Issues in the clinical management of intravenous drug users with HIV infection. *AIDS*, **3**, (Suppl 1), S201–S208.
14. Tong, T.G., Pond, S.M., Kreek, M.J., *et al.* (1981) Phenytoin induced methadone withdrawal. *Annals of Internal Medicine*, **90**, 361–72.
16. Gawin, F.H. & Ellinwood, E.H. (1988) Cocaine and other stimulants, actions, abuse and treatment. *New England Journal of Medicine*, **318**, 1173–82.
17. *Living with AIDS: a guide to survival by people with AIDS*. London: Frontliners.

Chapter 11

Death, Dying and Bereavement

Introduction

It has been commented that one of the most difficult aspects of HIV infection and AIDS is the unpredictability of how each individual will be affected. A person who seems to be profoundly ill may survive beyond all reasonable expectations. There is little predictability in the pattern of illness. Similarly with the grieving process. Many of the clients are young and have little previous experience of death amongst the people close to them. Similarly this can be true for the workers. Death remains among one of society's strongest taboos.

Grieving

When a person's appearance deteriorates as a result of HIV, grief and isolation can be further increased: Jeanette, for example, suffered from very severe facial dermatitis. She was acutely aware of this and told of incidents where she overheard children asking, 'What's wrong with that woman's face'. Her response to this was to stay at home on her own and drink.

There may be grief due to loss of involvement with children, relationships that break up, rejection from partners, family or friends: the client, for example, whose family bought him a 'special mug' when he told them he had been for a test (even though the result was negative). They kept the mug separate; no one else ever used it. It takes a considerable length of time to come to terms with the reality of HIV and AIDS and some clients never do. Nearly all IDUs will have known someone who has died as a result of their drug use, often as a result of unexpected overdose. They are less likely to be familiar with the progressive deterioration and disablement that HIV can cause. They are also subject to the uncertainties that arise when someone with HIV becomes desperately ill and then makes a recovery. IDUs will respond to death like everyone else in that their response will be individual.

According to Kubler-Ross[1], the process of loss can be seen as a series of 'stages'. There is great individual variation and adherence to the following sequence does not necessarily imply psychological health, nor does deviation from it imply pathology. People may not go through all of the stages; they may exhibit none of them, they may stick at particular stages or go back.[2]

(1) *Denial* ('not me'). Disbelief can be protective in allowing people time to adjust to their illness. There can be denial in an 'everyday' sense in that people can try to make the best of every day available to them, and continue to feel hope and enjoyment. It may mean pushing the issue to the back of their minds. It may also mean that they do not really succeed very well and it impinges on their thoughts a lot of the time. However, they may still be reluctant to talk about it with the worker. They may 'self-medicate' in an attempt to blot out unacceptable thoughts.

(2) *Anger* ('why me?'). Rage may be expressed towards significant others, and towards health care workers. In counselling and therapy people can be encouraged to express anger and identify its real target – death. Hostility to others may be used to hide the pain they feel about their lives.

(3) *Bargaining* ('yes me, but if only'). This occurs when people make bargains with God or fate, postponing the day of death by pretence or pleading – I promise to 'be good' until a certain event or date.

(4) *Depression* ('yes, me'). Here, there is deep experience of loss, with grieving and mourning over the changes that have occurred or will occur.

(5) *Acceptance* ('meaning attached to me'). This does not mean passive resignation, but the point when unfinished business (emotional and practical) has been handled, reality of death has been confronted (funeral planned; end of life imminent; willingness to let go of relationships; recognition of achievements, accomplishments; place of own life in 'greater order' [e.g. lives of others, influence on 'the world', position in the universe or with God/higher being]). Resolution and acceptance may be feasible only with clients who have a more stable lifestyle or who have managed to get some order into their lives. Some stages may be bypassed entirely, while others may last only a few minutes. Clients may want to attempt to make sense of AIDS. This may mean going over 'old ground' with them at intervals during the progression of their illness. If you want to check this out you can invite explanation by

asking the client if there is anything they need to know. Sometimes, as workers, we can get much too preoccupied with how we are coming across to be able to be sensitive to obvious cues in the client's behaviour. According to the AIDS Volunteers' Handbook, 'If we are uninvolved emotionally, it is easier to be sure that what we observe belongs to the bereaved'.[3] When the bereavement touches us it is easy to displace our own feelings onto others and to reach out and console ourselves in disguise.

Clients move around a lot and frequently see more than one worker. They may end up in hospitals other than the one they were initially treated at because of this. As a result, workers may only hear about the client's death some time later. The severe infections that clients can succumb to and their frequently intermittent medical care can contribute to the 'unfinished' feelings this can give rise to.

Talking about death

As death becomes imminent the client will spend more time sleeping and may be difficult to rouse. Encourage contact when the client is most alert. They may become disorientated and confused about the identity of those close and familiar to them. Reminders of day, time, who is in the room, etc. can help to reorient them. They may not be very responsive when death is near, but it is important that someone be with the client to reassure them. What most people fear is dying alone. When people are dying, they may simply need someone to *be with them* rather than to *do things* for them. A number of hospices provide an invaluable service in the provision of sensitive care for people in the terminal stages of AIDS. They can also provide support for their partners and families.

Putting affairs in order

This may be difficult to achieve with drug-using clients for the practical reasons that you may not be aware that the client has been taken into hospital or they may suddenly become very ill. The psychological barrier to preparing for death can be the client's strong denial of the reality of their situation.

Making a will

This is best done by a solicitor. Even if someone has very few possessions, they may have things they want given to people as keepsakes. If someone dies without leaving a will (intestate) their possessions will be divided amongst their nearest living relatives. If they are not married, then it is much easier for their partner to have provision made for them in a will, otherwise they will have to claim as a dependent and this can be difficult. If the client is concerned about becoming mentally incapable they can appoint someone with enduring power of attorney. This is especially important if the client is estranged from their family.

Living wills have recently been legalised in parts of Canada. These enable people to set out the conditions under which doctors should stop treatment. These wills are legally binding and federal legislation in Canada is proposed to protect doctors from criminal prosecution for following a patient's directives. The patient may want to talk to their doctor about issues such as resuscitation and mechanical ventilation; there is as yet no legislation for living wills in this country.

Funeral arrangements

If the client has specific wishes about funeral arrangements details of this can be put down in a will. At the very least they should write down what they want done and leave these instructions with someone they can rely on. They should let you know who they want notified of their death and, more importantly, who they want with them when they are about to die. A good undertaker can make a tremendous difference to the ease with which specific instructions can be carried out. Infectious diseases regulations will be imposed with varying degrees of stringency.

In Joe's family it was very important to have a wake: here, family and friends pay their respects to their dead relative who lies in a open coffin. The local Catholic priest was able to recommend an undertaker who was willing to consider this request. It also depends on the nursing staff and their level of experience in dealing with these deaths.

Families who cannot afford private funeral arrangements may have to have local authority funerals. Staff in hospitals who deal with patients' affairs will be familiar with these procedures and act swiftly, but if you are aware of any requests from the client regarding arrangements you should let the nursing staff know as soon as possible. Obviously if the client has to have a local authority-funded funeral then expenses will be kept to a minimum and thus choice will be limited. Financial assistance may be necessary if transport costs are involved and the bereaved cannot meet these. Unfortunately, charitable sources of financial assistance are limited. The bereaved, understandably, can be particularly distressed and chaotic at these times and arrangements may require extensive input on the part of the worker since it is unlikely that the client will have made plans prior to their death.

Families and partners

Where families are estranged from the IDU it is obviously a tremendous shock to inform them of their relative's death. They may also need to accept not only the loss, but also their relative's drug use. The client may have left instructions as to what information may or may not be disclosed after their death. There will be a need among some families to go over and over the events and memories of the deceased. Frequently idealisation of the person takes place. We need to be able to reassure people that their reactions to loss are 'normal' and include conflicting emotions: anger about leaving them; physical reactions; feeling that they are still around or that they came and talked to them. People should be reassured that there is no set time for them to 'get over it'. Bereaved partners of IDUs who also use drugs may relapse or go into a period of heavier drug use in order to cope with the pain and loss. I will never forget one funeral I attended of a client where most of the mourners were stoned out of their minds. We all have our own ways of coping; for the IDU this may include increased drug consumption. This can be a very dangerous time and it is crucial that they have some regular form of support. After a period of mourning, they may need to be encouraged to move on, establish new networks, new roles; sometimes they need to be given permission to get on with their lives. The worker can help them to discuss ambivalent feelings about their partner. They may also have to cope with fears for their own health and may experience increased physical symptoms, especially if they are antibody-positive. It is, of course, necessary not to dismiss these symptoms and to ensure they are checked in order to establish whether or not they are due to HIV or to stress, depression or anxiety. They may need help in order to say goodbye to the deceased. You can help them do this as sessions pass and continue to point out the changes that have taken place in their lives, the reduction in the symptoms of grief and guilt, and relief from physical aches and pains.

Family involvement

The IDU client often has difficult or non-existent communications with their family. There needs to be considerable commitment from both the client and their family if they want to be seen together. All parties need to attend willingly – dragging in reluctant participants is a waste of time. Due to attendance problems, often only brief interventions are possible.

Where family sessions are arranged they can provide a range of useful interventions and assist in reconciliation. They can also help with coming to terms with their partner's or relative's diagnosis and bereavement issues. In one example, the client had died of an overdose and the family wanted to get together to try to make sense of this. They had long since ceased to discuss the client's drug problems, trying to convince themselves that 'it was all under control'. After arguing about whether or not it was deliberate or an accident, they went on to express their guilt that they had not intervened sooner. The mother had felt all along that this would happen but had never been able to articulate this fear.

In a further example of this, one father who was informed that his son had been found dead in his squat, wanted us to confirm that his son had died of drug use rather than AIDS. As no postmortem took place, this was not possible to verify. His HIV-positive son had been quite ill but due to his chronic fear of going into hospital he had refused medical care, so there was no adequate information on his state of health. Initially the father had felt that it was more 'acceptable' for his son to have died of a drugs overdose than of AIDS. Everyone knew of his drug problem, but no one, apart from his father, knew of his HIV status. A double adjustment was required in coming to terms with HIV as well as the drug problem.

Some families or couples will have been putting a brave face on it for their relative because they do not want them to see how upset they are. This may lead them to reject any offer of help initially, but they may need it after their relative has died, so you should make it clear that you are available to see them, even if they should decide not to take up the offer for several weeks or months. Some of the issues they may want to discuss include the following:

- they may want to see you to talk about how to tell others of the result;
- there is frequently anger between family members about loss;
- if children are involved there can be enormous guilt and grief about children being infected;

- the worker can act as a mediator where there are unresolved relationships – this includes changes in the relationship as a result of illness, who is in control, who is now the more assertive and more organised;
- involvement in reaching a compromise regarding sexual activity;
- the provision of information and help to focus on quality of life rather than longevity.

Family work basically takes the form of facilitating communication between the individuals involved: finding out what their belief system is; providing appropriate information; and opening up the channels of communication to allow them to talk to each other, particularly where they are protecting each other from their worst fears. Frequently, allowing the family to express their concerns can come as an enormous relief.

There is a possibility that if you have been in the position of seeing a client individually and then expand your role to seeing the client's partner or family (even if this is at the client's request), this may lead to the client feeling resentful that they no longer have your exclusive support. If a specific therapeutic intervention is appropriate, then referral to a specialist, together with your 'behind the scenes' involvement, may be more appropriate.

Most families will be totally unfamiliar with the concept of airing their problems in public. They may also become overly dependent on the worker to 'sort things out': one mother, for example, whose son had been taken into prison, fought with the prison wardens because they would not let her give him the chicken she had cooked for him. She phoned the worker and asked if they would intervene for her by phoning the governor of the prison – 'he'll listen to you'. A problem of the use of the worker's time can emerge with families (as with individuals) who may try to enlist you to fight every battle on their behalf.

Some families will end up caring for the person with HIV or AIDS as they become increasingly ill. This can lead to relationship stresses within the family. The client may feel that their freedom is restricted, that they have to conform to rules that they left home to avoid. This may be particularly pertinent if the client wants to use non-prescribed drugs and the family object strongly to this.

Working with couples can be much more demanding than one to one work, but it can also be more constructive where the couple use the sessions to work out their relationship problems. Co-working when seeing couples has a number of important advantages: it increases the range of interventions; it can serve to prevent collusive relationships; the workers gain mutual supervision and support. Eliciting change where one member of the couple is a non-user is often easier than when both use. The bond of drug use is a particularly strong one. It can insulate the couple from other problems in their relationship and make it particularly difficult if one partner decides they want to change and the other does not. It is unusual for a relationship to survive if one partner becomes drug-free, particularly if the relationship developed when both partners were drug users. It is rare that both partners are totally in unison about what they want to do. Relationship breakdowns are traumatic emotionally and can have practical and financial implications. It is not surprising that attempts are made to maintain the status quo. Carers who are drug users themselves can find it particularly tough to admit that they are having difficulty coping. The situation can break down very easily and emergency access to respite care and community support is particularly necessary. In these cases the situation is frequently exacerbated by poor living conditions.

References

1. Kubler-Ross, E. (1977) *On death and dying*. London: Tavistock.
2. George, H. (1990) Coping with dying and bereavement. Course notes, Association for Psychological Therapies, Leicester.
3. *Volunteers' Handbook* (1985) Gay men's health crisis, New York.

Chapter 12

Education and Health Promotion

Introduction

The 'it won't happen to me' principle applies to drug users just as much as to any one else. In one study researchers compared drug clinic attenders' and students' responses to the government's AIDS education and drug use campaign. The drug users' perception of personal risk for AIDS was low: 42% of users and 24% of students felt that they personally were not at risk. Seeing the adverts did not increase drug users' anxiety levels. Most of them reported that they had not changed their injecting or sexual behaviour as a result of the education campaigns.[1]

According to Stockdale,[2] a new range of posters promoting a positive image to safer sex evoked a better response from heterosexuals. These posters are more sexually explicit and conveyed the idea that safer sex is 'trendy, does not interfere with love, and is practised by attractive people'. According to Stockdale, in order to succeed 'posters must stimulate our awareness, make us question our beliefs, and supply new, positive directions for our social (that of self perceptions) and behavioural repertoires'.

The 'just say no' message of much anti-drugs public education is an interesting one. I am reminded of a trip to Devon made by a team of drug workers for a 'team building' weekend. One piece of advice that was given was to avoid the local bitter as it induced certain brain death in all those foolhardy enough to try it. On visiting the local pub, all but one drug worker specifically asked for the brand of bitter they were advised not to touch!

Early in this century educational films were produced to try to prevent the spread of syphilis in US soldiers. These films used fear arousal messages and the finding was that fear was increased but behaviour did not change.[3] During World War 2, condoms and treatment for venereal diseases were made available and soldiers responded favourably. As many as 50 million condoms were accepted by soldiers each month and reports of syphilis incidence decreased in this population over time.[4]

Knowledge does not necessarily change behaviours, nor do messages that have a fear arousing content. Ideally, the combination should emphasise an individual's ability to respond or change and also individualise his or her perception of the threat. In this way, the individual sees that the threat exists for them personally, but that they are in a position to do something about it. We need to know what community norms have meaning for the drug user – are they already an 'out group', stigmatised as a result of their drug use? Does a strong sense of community exist for the IDU? What effect does the illegality of drug use have on this? These are all questions that have not yet received adequate attention.

Perceptions of risk

An individual who believes an outcome is inevitable will be reluctant to undertake difficult changes in behaviour. The minimum requirements for behaviour change are that the individual perceives themselves to be at risk. Many IDUs have already changed their injecting behaviour and therefore have a lowered perception of risk,[5,6] that is, they have already reduced the risk that they identify with – syringe sharing. A far greater emphasis is needed on sexual transmission; this means identifying with a possibly weaker peer group – heterosexuals in general rather than drug users in particular – with a dilution in the strength of the response. Among respondents to a recent national telephone survey in the US, those who reported five or more sexual partners in the last year indicated that they had never purchased condoms during that time. IDUs may simply be conforming to community norms – deviation from these norms may increase stigmatisation for them.[3]

Initiating change

In order for change to occur, social and behavioural science offers some guidance.[3] The following points should be borne in mind:

- people must be motivated, believe that the change will do some good, and believe that they have a reasonable chance of accomplishing it;
- it should also be consistent with the individual's beliefs and values;

- people need assistance and support in order to change and many will not be completely successful in adhering to new behaviour patterns;
- it is often easier to get people to modify a behaviour than to eliminate it;
- encourage incremental behaviour changes rather than global lifestyle changes. 'Instead of looking at what has to change, let us look at what can stay the same.'[3]
- offer choices among alternative behaviours rather than rigidly presenting a single behaviour. Options and choices encourage a motivated response;

In San Francisco workers have found that for community change to be successful it requires the following measures:

(1) Strong leadership.
(2) Market research.
(3) An informed and motivated target audience.
(4) Activities to facilitate change.
(5) Use of multiple channels of communication.
(6) Grass roots participation.

The cultural context is also important. One creative approach to this was undertaken is Santa Domingo amongst Haitian–Creole workers (who were predominantly Roman Catholic). They had an annual collective baptism of the condom during their Easter celebrations. This was done to condone condom use as a culturally acceptable behaviour. This, plus other public education efforts, led to an increased AIDS awareness and significant increase in condom use in the community.[7] Where IDUs are concerned, we need to overome the following:

(1) Popular mythologies such as attitudes towards condoms – myths that need to be dispelled because they are a barrier to change.
(2) The problem with the time lag between the behaviour and the adverse outcome – much of the drug use behaviour is based on immediate gratification.
(3) The fatalism or apathy which we see in some clients. 'AIDS is just one more risk for drug users' 43% of respondents agreed.[5] I am reminded of the comment of one HIV-positive woman, 'if I had to choose between a drug problem and HIV, I'd choose HIV every time. At least you can forget about it. I don't have to cope with feelings of craving where HIV is concerned'.

(4) Poor access to health care.
(5) Stigmatisation of drug users.

A number of theoretical explanations and models exist to attempt to elucidate the factors that determine why we do or do not change our behaviour. There have always been benefits for not sharing syringes prior to HIV. Clients who did not share before HIV often reported fear of hepatitis and other health problems as a reason for not sharing. The physical benefits of sharp new needles are also obvious since they will prolong the longevity of veins. Simple increased availability, therefore, is likely to be taken advantage of.

Safe sex guidelines recommend (among other things) the use of condoms with the benefits of contraception and protection against STDs. However, the barriers to condom use extend far beyond availability.[8] Many of the clients believe that condoms fail regularly. What is the point of going to all that trouble if the condom is going to fail anyway? Perceived susceptibility is also considered relevant. The possible consequences of not using a condom are very far removed as far as HIV is concerned, whereas the discomfort of injecting with a blunt needle is fairly readily apparent. Self efficacy or belief in one's ability to perform a behaviour is a major factor in success. Self efficacy is generally low among IDUs.

According to Becker, a combination of self-efficacy, value of health, availability, normative beliefs (i.e. condoms spoil sex), and response efficacy (i.e. taking the action that will be worthwhile), all contribute in accounting for behaviour change or lack of it.[9]

Rogers' protection – motivation theory,[10] is one of the few that considers coping on an interpersonal level, that is, with the other person. Where condom use is concerned, two people (at least) are involved. There are also cultural, economic, religious and political factors to consider, in other words models must transcend the individual.

Caroline Cupitt, the researcher at St Mary's, has come up with her own formulation to account for behaviour change among drug users.

(1) *Threat* – severity of problem; perceived vulnerability to problem.
(2) *Coping* – self-efficacy and response-efficacy.
(3) *Cost* – response cost
    (a) negotiation
    (b) normative views
    (c) infertility (perceived or actual)
    (d) availability/finance
(4) *Situation-specific variables*

(a) effect of drugs taken
(b) availability of/or drugs taken
(c) mood
(d) negotiation
(e) contraceptive needs

In the counselling setting the significance of each of these variables can be assessed for the individual and interventions tailored to meet their needs. Every stage will be coloured by the IDUs previous experience. The model is totally interactive. Different areas are defined for the purposes of the model and not all these boundaries will exist in real life situations.

According to Bandura,[11] a person's ability is not necessarily based on past performance. One's perceived ability to execute specific behaviours can, therefore, be moulded. If we can help the client build up a sense of self-competency and the necessary skills to carry them out effectively, then we can improve self-efficacy.

Peer education

Leaflets at best only inform, however well they are produced. Information and improved attitudes are not necessarily translated into action. Also, limitations on vocabulary and reading ability will be an impediment to understanding HIV prevention messages.

It is very reinforcing to see someone similar to us who can change[12] and one of the strongest predictors of behaviour change is the participation of friends in risk-reduction activities. Peer educators and opinion leaders among IDUs could be used to disseminate educational messages. When the ideas are new, the source of information must be credible. A worker in a syringe exchange remarked recently that he was fed up hearing the clients comment that, 'Jimi Hendrix was a real good bloke'. If he were alive today, perhaps he could have helped.

In New York ex-users are employed as outreach workers who give information about syringe cleaning and offer HIV counselling and access to testing. In one study the reported mean monthly injection rate decreased from 34 at baseline to 10 at follow-up ($p < 0.0001$; 140 median days to follow-up); 53% reported using condoms at least once over the study period as opposed to 36% at baseline ($p < 0.05$).[13] However, other studies in the USA have found that although there were decreases in drug-related activities, there was no comparable reduction in sexual risk practices.[14]

In one study in San Francisco, knowledge gains measured shortly after an educational programme in a residential drug treatment unit disappeared over the next six months; self-efficacy, however, was increased following the intervention ($p = 0.07$) and significantly enhanced at six-month follow-up ($p = 0.02$).[15] This highlights the importance of repeated efforts at training and education. If training can increase self-efficacy, and this is sustained, then it will be helpful to the individual in instituting and sustaining behaviour change in the future.

Imaginative methods of skills training have also been investigated. In 'Bartenders Against AIDS' in San Francisco, information on HIV prevention was given to local bartenders; this included training on how to promote the message of safer sex among customers. An interesting strategy was used by Schilling *et al.*[16] Drug workers used skills-building training methods with women who were on a methadone programme. In the first two sessions they provided information on AIDS and HIV-prevention through video, visual presentation, and didactic group exercises designed to enable participants to identify their own high risk sexual behaviour and discuss the barriers to adopting safer sex.

In the third session they discussed the negative associations of condoms, practised rolling condoms on to demonstration models, and role-played different scenarios where partners were asked to use condoms.

In the fourth and fifth sessions they participated in assertiveness training, problem solving and communication skills in modelled scenarios involving safer sex. They practised skills by first scripting scenarios and then personalised the skills by role playing scenarios that reflected their own lives.

Compared with the controls in an information giving only group, the skills-building group reported that they felt more comfortable discussing safer sex with their partners and both carried and used condoms more frequently.

Skills need to be fostered, rehearsed and reinforced in order for them to be transferred into practice. Training sessions require repetition, a variety of teaching styles, and feedback to enable clients to express their fears.

A number of self-help organisations for IDUs already exist, the Junkibonden, for instance, in Amsterdam, and ADAPT in New York. Similar organisations (for example, Mainliners) have been developed for users and ex-users in the United Kingdom. An increasing number of drug agencies encourage local support group initiatives such as users groups at syringe exchange units.

Setting up support groups can take a lot of energy on the part of the facilitator and are not easily sustained. Erratic attendance, with occasionally more staff than clients, can prove disheartening at times. However, if maintenance of the group is seen as the job of the agency as a whole and not the sole responsibility of a few committed individuals, especially if time for the group is part of the unit's daily routine, then the pressure can be relieved somewhat. The group should provide a safe place for the sharing of experiences and allow a forum for information-giving and the development of a peer network. The IDU may choose to attend the group erratically, as and when the need arises. A number of HIV-positive clients have also looked on support groups as places to meet someone in the same position as themselves. Ideally, the client should not leave the group feeling worse than when they arrived.

The role of the group facilitator is just that, they should be prepared to facilitate communication between members of the group and try to see that each person gets adequate opportunities to give and get attention (although this can in fact be difficult to realise). The facilitator needs to avoid moral posturing and also to resist the temptation to set up a 'therapy group'. He or she should be prepared to digress with the group when a subject arouses general interest or feelings. Invited speakers may occasionally be used to discuss specialist issues but they should be warned of the possibility of a poor turnout. Spector and Conklin[17] found that it was essential that the facilitator be as knowledgeable as possible, particularly on aspects of HIV, since clients continually bring information to the group for validation or clarification.

At the support groups for drug users and ex-users held at the Terrence Higgins Trust (THT), it was anticipated that mixing users, ex-users and scripted clients might have been difficult due to their differing aims and needs, but this did not in fact turn out to be the case. They found that, 'the ex-users tend to be a positive influence on the others in terms of generating motivation to come off drugs, as well as being generally supportive to each other'.[18] What they did find to be a more significant factor was mixing clients at different stages of HIV disease in the same group. Spector and Conklin found it a more viable proposition if the group were composed of people at similar stages of the disease. The presence of very debilitated people induced fear in those who were asymptomatic, as well as guilt for being well.

Same-gender groups have been found to be an appropriate intervention for women in the drug treatment setting. Whereas gender or sexual preference can be a fairly straightforward way of grouping clients, specifying who the group is and is not intended for can sometimes go to extremes. One bewildered person with AIDS commented, 'Soon they'll be having support groups for the pets of people with AIDS'.

The subjects that were of interest in the THT drugs users support group were found to be the following:

(1) Access to grants for furniture, travel, outstanding bills, clothing, telephones, emergency accommodation.
(2) Access to information about HIV treatments, drug treatments, sympathetic agencies.
(3) Social support for overcoming isolation, facing fears, breaking taboos, meeting prospective partners, exchanging ideas, generating further support networks.
(4) Emotional support – safe environment, working through unfinished business, lifeline.
(5) Access to medical facilities for primary health, contraception, condoms, etc.; advice about needle exchange.
(6) Access to drug treatment – referral to prescribing agencies.[18]

Some of the more creative approaches to stimulating discussion on safer sex issues in support groups have involved enlisting the help of actors from AIDS-based theatre groups who act out vignettes relevant to the group members; group members can then discuss this without feeling the subject to be too personal or threatening. Treatment approaches that consider alternatives to abstinence from drugs are also being more widely used.

Relapse prevention is a skills-based therapy package which takes account of high-risk situations and has wide applications in the risk-reduction context. It trains people that, 'one lapse does not a failure make', and combines skills training and cognitive interventions – the client and worker re-think the skills necessary to resist a risk-associated activity and use relapse action planning and behavioural contracting and rehearsal. It is designed for the control of indulgent behaviours that require immediate gratification and are followed by delayed negative consequences. The length of intervention is an important factor: length of treatment, the method of learning skills and training in relapse rehearsal can lead to increased perception of self-efficacy and decrease the probability of relapse.[19]

Motivational milieu therapy attempts to meet the needs of the unmotivated client. Counselling interventions encourage the client to change when they see their drug-taking behaviour as incompatible with their view of themselves or their feelings about what they should be like or should be doing.[20] The treatment philosophy holds that change progresses along a certain phase structure: motivation for change is not a personal trait and can be influenced in the interaction between client and therapist; controlled drug use is possible. A supportive environment will ensure a quicker adoption and more consistent maintenance of the behaviour change. However, a combination of approaches, an awareness of context – the availability of condoms, for example, peer educators, leaflets, TV, adverts, posters, and skills-based training) – will all enhance the likelihood of behaviour change.

References

1. Sherr, L. (1990) Fear arousal and AIDS. *AIDS*, **4**, (4), 354–61.
2. Stockdale, J. (1990) In Coughlan A. Postive posters make the AIDS message stick. *New Scientist*, August 20th.
3. Turner, C.F., Miller, H.G. & Moses, L.E. (1989) *Sexual behaviour and intravenous drug use*. Washington DC: National Academy Press.
4. Lashley, K.S. & Watson, J.B. (1922) *A psychological study of motion pictures in relation to venereal disease campaigns*. US Interdepartmental Social Hygiene Board, Washington DC.
5. Mulleady, G., White, D., Phillips, K. & Cupitt, C. (1990) Reducing sexual transmission of HIV for injecting drug users: the challenge for counselling. *Counselling Psychology Quarterly*, **3**, (4), 325–41.
6. Stimson, G.V., Alldritt, L., Dolan, K.A., Donoghue, M.C. & Hart, R. (1988) Injecting equipment exchange schemes. Final report. Monitoring Research Group. Goldsmiths' College, London.
7. Didiez, N., Arbaje, M., & Rosario, S., *et al.* (1989) The gaga baptism of the condom: folklore and religion as adjuncts of AIDS prevention among Haitian migrant agricultural workers in the Dominican Republic. V International Conference on AIDS, Montreal (Abstract MEO 11).
8. Cupitt, C., Mulleady, G., White, D. & Phillips, K. (1991) Sexual behaviour change in IVDUs. Unpublished manuscript.
9. Becker, M. (1974) The health belief modes and personal health behaviour. *Health Education Monograph*, **2**, 328–85.
10. Rogers, R.W. (1975) A protection motivation theory of fear appeals and attitude change. *The Journal of Psychology*, **91**, 93–114.
11. Bandura, A. (1989) Perceived self efficacy in the exercise of personal agency. *The Psychologist*, October **1**, 989, 411–24.
12. Friedman, S.R., Des Jarlais, D.C., Southeran, J.L., Garber, J., Cohen H. & Smither, D. (1987) AIDS and self organisation among intravenous drug users. *International Journal of the Addictions*, **22**, 201–19.
13. Sufian, M., Friedman, S.R., Neaigus, A., Goldsmith, D., Des Jarlais, D.E. & Graves, F. (1989) Risk reduction after outreach intervention among intravenous drug users. V International Conference on AIDS, Montreal (Abstract WEP 68).

14. Jain, S., Flynn, N., Bailey, V., Sweha, A., Ding, D. & Sloan, E. (1989) IVDU and AIDS: more resistance to changing their sexual than their needle sharing practices. V International Conference on AIDS. Montreal (Abstract WDP 79).
15. Sorenson, J.L., Gibson, D.R., Heitzman, D., Dumontet, R. & Constantini, M. (1989) Psychoeducational group approach to AIDS prevention with drug abusers in residential treatment: impact six months after intervention. V International Conference on AIDS, Montreal (Abstract ThDP 84).
16. Schilling, R.F., El-Bassel, N., Schinke, S.P., Gordon, K. & Nichols, S. (1991) Reducing sexual transmission of AIDS: skills building with recovering female drug users. Public Health Reports. (In press.)
17. Spector, J. & Conklin, R. (1987) AIDS group psychotherapy. *International Journal of Group Psychotherapy*, **37**, 433–9.
18. Hogarth, S. (1988) Support group for drug users with HIV, ARC, AIDS: history and guidelines. Drugs Education Group, Terrence Higgins Trust, London.
19. Marlatt, G.A. & George, W. (1984) Relapse prevention: introduction and overview of the model. *British Journal of Addiction*, **79**, 261–73.
20. Van Bilsen, H.P.J.G. (1986) Heroin addiction: morals revisited. *Journal of Substance Abuse Treatment*, **3**, 279–84.

Resources

HIV, AIDS and AIDS-related drugs services

Aids and Housing Project
Write for information to 16–18 Strutton Ground, London SW1 2HP.

Aids Ahead
A consortium of AIDS organisations for deaf people and the hard of hearing. Informal advice, counselling and interpreters.
38 Victoria Place, Carlisle, Cumbria.
Vistel: 0228 28719; Voice: 0228 4994.

Association Française d'Aide aux Seropositifs (AFAS+)
Offers a telephone hotline giving advice, support and information about HIV and AIDS to French-speaking people.
Tel: 071 383 0489, Mon–Thu 7 pm–10 pm; Tue 2 pm–4 pm.

Blackliners
Helpline for black people concerned about HIV and AIDS.
PO Box 1274, London SW9 3EZ.
Helpline tel: 071 738 5274, Mon–Fri 9 am–5 pm.

Black HIV and AIDS Network
106–108 King Street, Hammersmith, London W6.
Contact National AIDS Helpline (below) for telephone number.

Body Positive
Mutual help and support groups for people with HIV. For address and phone number of local group, phone the National AIDS Helpline (0800 567 123) or Body Positive, London (below). The London Centre also offers free legal advice by Immunity Legal Centre (6 pm–8 pm.)
Write or drop in: 51 Philbeach Gardens, London SW5 9EB.
Helpline tel: 071 373 9124, daily 7 pm–10 pm.

Body Positive Women's Core Group
National group which meets monthly at Body Positive Centre in London to provide mutual support and plan women's responses to HIV and AIDS. For information and membership details write to Body Positive, London (above).
Tel: 071 835 1045.

Care and Resources for People Affected by HIV and AIDS (CARA)
Christian group offering support to Christians and non-Christians affected by HIV and AIDS.
178 Lancaster Road, London W11 1QU.
Tel: 071 792 8299.

Crusaid
A fund-raising organisation which helps people with AIDS in need of practical and financial assistance.
83 Clerkenwell Road, London EC1R 5AR.
Tel: 071 831 2595/8.

Dublin AIDS Alliance
Cairde
Irish Frontliners
Body Positive (Dublin)
Women and AIDS
Organisations offering advice and support about HIV and AIDS for people in Ireland.
189–193 Avoca House, Parrell Street, Dublin 1.

Foundation for AIDS Counselling Treatment and Support
Provides a GP service, counselling and complimentary health services and training for health care workers.
Weston Park, Crouch End, London N8 9SY.
Tel: 081 348 9195.

Gay Bereavement Project
Telephone support and advice for those bereaved by the death of a same sex partner.
Tel: 081 455 8894.

Immunity Legal Centre
Specialist legal and welfare rights advice centre for people in the Greater London area who have legal problems associated with HIV and

AIDS. Produces an information booklet on HIV and the law. Offers sessions at Body Positive Drop-In Centre, London Lighthouse, and the Landmark.
260a Kilburn Lane, London W10.
Tel: 081 969 8909, Mon–Fri, 10 am–5 pm.

Jewish AIDS Trust
Offers support, education, counselling, practical help and referrals to people in Jewish community who are affected by HIV and AIDS.
PO Box 799, London N3.
Tel: 081 455 6449.

Landmark
Day centre for people with HIV or AIDS.
Mon and Thu, 10 am–9 pm; Tue and Fri, 10 am–5 pm; Wed, 10 am–7 pm. Women-only evening, Wed 7 pm–9 pm.
47a Tulse Hill, London SW2.
Tel: 081 671 7611.

London Lesbian and Gay Switchboard
24-hour advice and information service.
BM Switchboard, London WC1N 3XX.
Tel: 071 837 7324.

London Lighthouse
Residential and support centre for people affected by HIV and AIDS. Counselling, support groups, creative and complementary therapies, home support, respite, convalescence and terminal care.
111–117 Lancaster Road, London W11 1QT.
Tel: 071 792 1200.

Mainliners
Support, advice and help for those with, or at risk of, HIV or AIDs who use, or have used, drugs (illegal and legal).
PO Box 125, London SW9 8EF.
Helpline tel: 071-737 3141.
Office/administration: 071-274 4000, extension 315.

Mildmay Mission Hospital
Convalescence, respite and terminal care. Has mother and baby rooms. Covers City and East London.
Hackney Road, London E2 7NA.
Tel: 071 729 2331.

National AIDS Helpline
24-hour advice and information service.
(All calls are free and are not listed on itemised phone bills.)
Tel: 0800 567 123.
For leaflets:
Tel: 0800 555 777 24-hour service.
Bengali, Gujerati, Hindi, Punjabi, Urdu Helpline:
Tel: 0800 282 445, Wed 6 pm–10 pm.
Cantonese Helpline:
Tel: 0800 282 446 Tue 6 pm–10 pm.
Arabic Helpline:
Tel: 0800 282 447, Wed 6 pm–10 pm.
Minicom terminal for the hard of hearing:
Tel: 0800 521 361, daily 10 am–10 pm.

National Association of Citizens' Advice Bureaux, HIV Project
Provides education, information, resources, training and counselling.
115–123 Pentonville Road, London N1 9LZ.
Tel: 071 833 2181.

National Freephone (recorded information: all calls are free)
Arabic tel: 0800 622 507
Bengali tel: 0800 622 501
Cantonese tel: 0800 622 506
English tel: 0800 622 509
Gujerati tel: 0800 622 503
Hindi tel: 0800 622 502
Punjabi tel: 0800 622 504
Urdu tel: 0800 622 505.

Nurses' Support Group
For nurses needing support and advice with HIV and related problems.
Tel: 071 708 5605 (Mon and Wed 7 pm–10 pm.)

Positively Irish Action on AIDS
21 Old Ford Road, London, E2 9PL.
Tel: 081 983 0192.

Positive Partners/Positively Children
Offers support groups, helpline, training, advice, information and support for people who are HIV-positive and their partners and families.
Manor Gardens Centre, 8 Manor Gardens, London N7 6LA.

Tel: 071 272 4231 (also daytime helpline).
071 239 6068 (evening helpline).

Positively Women
Women offering support, counselling and information to women with HIV or AIDS.
5 Sebastian Street, London EC1V 0HE.
Tel: 071 490 5515, 9.30 am–5.30 pm.
Office/administration tel: 071-490 5501.

Project for Advice, Counselling and Education (PACE)
Offers free individual, couple and group counselling and a weekly clinic for one-off crisis counselling, by appointment.
London Lesbian and Gay Centre, 67–69 Lowcross Street, London EC1M 6BP.
Tel: 071 251 2689.

Scottish AIDS Monitor
Advice and information about HIV and AIDS for people in Scotland.
PO Box 169, Edinburgh EH1 3UU.
Tel: 031 588 1167, Mon–Fri 7.30 pm–10 pm.

St Mungo Family Life AIDS Groups (FLAGS)
Offers accommodation to people with AIDS in safe, secure and supportive homes, where each person can live as full and independent a life as possible.
Flags Coordinator, St Mungo Community Trust, Bishop Creighton House, 378 Lillie Road, London SW6.
Tel: 071 381 6680.

Terrence Higgins Trust
Provides information, advice and help on HIV and AIDS. Produces specific information on AIDS for gay men, drug users, women and lesbians. Offers counselling, prison visiting, support groups and home support. Also has a 'hardship fund'.
52–54 Grays Inn Road, London WC1X 8JU.
Helpline tel: 071 242 1010, 3 pm–10 pm.
Legal line tel: 071 405 2381, Wed 7 pm–10 pm.
Office/administration tel: 071 831 0330.

Threshold Housing Advice Centre
Advice for people who are affected by HIV/AIDS who are homeless or

face a housing problem.
126 Uxbridge Road, London W12.
Tel: 081-749 2925.

Drugs services

Adfam
Advice and support for families of drug users.
Unit 7, South Thames Studios, 511 Lavington Street, London SE1 0NZ.
Tel: 071 401 2079.

Alcohol Concern
A national organisation with advice and information about local services.
305 Grays Inn Road, London WC1X 8QF.
Tel: 081-833 3471.

Drugs, Alcohol, Women, Nationally (DAWN)
Advice and information for women with drugs or alcohol problems.
Produces information leaflets/booklets. Omnibus workspace.
39–41 North Road, London N7 9DP.
Tel: 071-700 4653 (24-hour answerphone).

Families Anonymous
Advice and support for the families and friends of drug users.
Linked with Narcotics Anonymous.
5–7 Parsons Green, London SW6 4UL.
Helpline tel: 071 731 8060.

Institute for the Study of Drug Dependence (ISDD)
Britain's national information service on the misuse of drugs.
Has a library and book mailing service.
1 Hatton Place, London EC1N 8ND.
Tel: 071 430 1993.

Narcotics Anonymous
Self-help groups for people dependent on drugs.
PO Box 246, c/o 47 Milman's Street, London SW10.
Tel: 071 351 6794/6066 (24-hour answerphone).

Release
Provides information and advice on drug-related problems, including legal problems.
169 Commercial Street, London E1 6BW.
Advice Line tel: 071-377 5905 (10 am–6 pm).
Emergencies only tel: 071-603 8654.

Scottish Drug Forum
Similar function to SCODA (below) for Scottish agencies.
266 Clyde Street, Glasgow, G1 4JH.
Tel: 041 221 1175.

Standing Conference on Drug Abuse (SCODA)
Comprehensive library and information service on drug problems and services.
HIV/AIDS information officer can provide an up-to-date list of syringe exchange facilities nationally.
1–4 Hatton Place, London EC1N 8RU.
Tel: 071 430 2341/3.

Other services and support organisations

Association of British Insurers
Advice on insurance problems.
Tel: 071 248 4477.

British Pregnancy Advisory Service
Provides counselling help with abortion and artificial insemination and has branches in many parts of the country (see telephone directory for local organisations).
Austy Manor, Wooton Wawen, Solihull, West Midlands B95 6BX.
Tel: 0564 793 225.

Community Health Councils (CHC)
Advice on local health services and support in complaining about the service you received.
See telephone directory for local office.

Haemophilia Society
123 Westminster Bridge Road, London SE1 7HR.
Tel: 071 928 2020.

Health Education Authority
Provides advice, access to resources, and general information.
Hamilton House, Mabledon Place, London WC1H 9TX.
Tel: 071 383 3833.

Medical Advisory Services for Travellers Abroad
Keppel Street, London WC1.
Tel: 071 831 5333 (recorded message).

Organisation for Parents Under Stress (OPUS)
106 Godstone Road, Whyteleafe, Surrey CR3 0EB.
Tel: 081 645 0469.
Nottingham 24-hour crisis line tel: 0602 470551.

Rape Crisis
London centre offers 24-hour answerphone and can put you in touch with your nearest service.
PO Box 69, London WC1.
Tel: 071 837 1600.

Women's Health Information Centre and Women's Reproductive Rights Campaign (WHRRIC)
Advice for women on health and reproductive issues including HIV infection and AIDS.
52 Featherstone Street, London WC1Y 8RT.
Tel: 071-271 6332/6580.

Alternative and complementary therapies

There are numerous types of alternative therapies available. You will need to find out what suits you and find a reputable practitioner. Personal recommendation is valuable. The following organisations may be able to offer help and advice:

British Holistic Medical Association
179 Gloucester Place, London NW1 6DX.
Tel: 071 262 5299.

British Homoeopathic Association
27a Devonshire Street, London W1N 1RJ.
Tel: 071 935 2163.

Confederation of Healing Organisations (Greater London)
Tel: 071 735 2654.

Holistic AIDS Research Trust (HART)
BMHART, London WC1N 3XX.
Tel: 081 693 4812 (evenings); 0273 698698 (daytime).

Float Experience
South West London area. The Float Tank Association is run from this number. Contact for details of local floatation tanks.
Tel: 071 350 1001 (24-hour answerphone).

Institute for Complementary Medicine
21 Portland Place, London W1N 3AF.
Tel: 071 636 9543.

London Buddhist Centre
This centre teaches two meditation techniques. Free introductory sessions every Wednesday from 7 pm–9.30 pm. Six-week courses take place in Covent Garden, London.
Tel: 081-981 1225.

Natural Health Network
Chardstock House, Chard, Somerset, TA20 2TL.
Tel: 04606 3229.

Sivanda Yoga Centre
51 Felsham Road, London SW15.
Tel: 081 780 0160.

Society for Teachers of the Alexander Technique
Send SAE for details of your nearest practitioner.
10 London House, 266 Fulham Road, London SW10.
Tel: 071 351 0828.

Journals and newsletters

Several of the organisations already mentioned produce regular newsletters.

Body Positive newsletter called 'BP Newsletter'.
Mainliners newsletter called 'Mainliners Newsletter'.

There are a wide variety of journals available. Some use what may be difficult scientific terminology, some provide summary information. It can be useful to look at back copies to see if they are suitable to your needs. A number of specialist drug journals regularly carry articles on HIV, AIDS and drug issues, e.g. the *British Journal of Addiction*, *Druglink*, the *Journal of Psychoactive Drugs*.

Leading scientific journals include the following:

AIDS Newsletter
Brief summaries of current information on HIV and AIDS. Updated monthly.

AIDS
An international bi-monthly journal. Covers scientific research on HIV/AIDS.

British Medical Journal
Up-to-date articles on medical/scientific issues. Regularly includes articles on HIV/AIDS. Weekly.

Journal of the American Medical Association
Covers articles/issues on HIV/AIDS. Includes a section on the CDC morbidity and mortality report (MMWR). Weekly.

The Lancet
Similar to the BMJ (above). Good preliminary research reports. Weekly.

Nature
Includes general information on HIV/AIDS. Weekly.

New Scientist
Has a section called the 'AIDS Monitor'; covers issues relating to HIV/AIDS. Weekly.

New England Journal of Medicine
Includes results of some of the longer term studies in the USA on HIV/AIDS progression and treatment. Weekly.

Index